OLIVER HUCKEL

MENTAL MEDICINE

SOME PRACTICAL SUGGESTIONS FROM A SPIRITUAL STANDPOINT

WITH AN INTRODUCTION BY
LEWELLYS F. BARKER

Elibron Classics
www.elibron.com

Elibron Classics series.

ISBN 1-4021-6606-0 (paperback)
ISBN 1-4212-8161-9 (hardcover)

This Elibron Classics Replica Edition is an unabridged facsimile of the edition published in 1909 by Thomas Y. Crowell & Co., New York.

MENTAL MEDICINE

BY OLIVER HUCKEL, S. T. D.

MENTAL MEDICINE

SOME PRACTICAL SUGGESTIONS
FROM A SPIRITUAL STANDPOINT

Five Conferences with Students at the Johns Hopkins Medical School, by

OLIVER HUCKEL, S. T. D.

Graduate, University of Pennsylvania
Student at Oxford and Berlin Universities
Pastor, Associate Congregational Church, Baltimore

With an Introduction by
LEWELLYS F. BARKER, M. D.
Professor of Medicine in Johns Hopkins University

NEW YORK
THOMAS Y. CROWELL & CO.
PUBLISHERS

Published, June, 1909

CONTENTS

AUTHOR'S FOREWORD

THE introduction which Dr. Lewellys F. Barker of Johns Hopkins University has kindly written for this volume shows most clearly the scope and purpose of these addresses. I feel that his words may also do a great deal towards straightening out the tangled ideas of many regarding the relations of the differing professions of the physician and the clergyman in their mutual ministry to the "sick mind."

In addition to Dr. Barker's words, it seems fitting that a few words should be said from the standpoint of my own profession.

These present days are witnessing numerous attempts at closer co-operation between the physician and the minister in the processes of health and healing. There are also some endeavors to readjust the church as a universal hospital and clinic for the cure of certain forms of disease, while the clergy, in some instances are giving the bulk of their ministry to the art of healing by psychotherapeutic methods, including much of hypnotism.

We believe that the church will be wise in making haste slowly in the attempt at healing. There is real danger of giving itself, not to wise and rational psychotherapy, but to the extravagances of psychotherapeutic theories. It would be a distinct calamity if every church should be exploiting itself as a nervine hospital. There are also grave ethical dangers in the use of hypnotism.

Is there not possible, however, a wiser co-operation, and a safe and sane method? The addresses in this volume, in their spirit and teaching, endeavor to indicate what many of us believe to be the better way. They give a series of teaching along the lines of right thinking and right living, which ought to help make better conditions for health and healing. They eschew hypnotism. They aim to suggest a method of co-operation which can be readily used by all the churches, even if they do not have in their pulpit a trained psychologist, or in their equipment the necessary helpers for a church clinic. For most churches, this limited co-operation is all that is needed or advisable.

These addresses aim to incorporate the

fundamental teachings of mental science as used in modern psychotherapy. They do not exaggerate mental and spiritual factors. They do not make rash promises. They do not minimize the regular therapeutic methods, approved by long experience and fruitful results. They do not, for a moment, take the place of the physician. Rather, they aim to co-operate cordially and to make the physician's work more effective by supplementing it with certain mental and spiritual factors, which religious teaching can often most helpfully supply.

The writer feels that nothing final is said in these lectures. They are only tentative. Others will yet do fuller and better work. But up to the present, perhaps there is no book which fills just this field or meets this need, which is that of practical suggestion and present service along vital lines.

These addresses were given during February and March, 1909, in conference with students at the Johns Hopkins Medical School, under the auspices of the Medical Y. M. C. A., as an illustration of the new suggestive thought of the physical aspects of spiritual work, and also as a concrete exposition of how a minister's teaching might co-ordinate with and supplement the work of the physician. I have been surprised and gratified at the cordial reception these addresses have already received, and the large usefulness they have demonstrated, as witnessed by the spoken testimonies and many letters. I hope that in their printed form they may be equally serviceable.

These addresses, being given under the auspices of the Young Men's Christian Association of the Medical School of the University, have allowed me to emphasize the spiritual aspect of these matters much more strongly than I would otherwise have taken the liberty of doing. Under these auspices I felt that my work was not merely to discuss theories, but in a definite sense to help create a spiritual atmosphere, leading to some practical results, even among the students themselves. If these addresses, therefore, shall have any value to the public, it ought to be along these lines. They are not medical lectures; they are vital discussions for immediate inspiration and helpfulness.

Some needed notes of warning are being sounded in these days against the interest of ministers in psychotherapy, and some admirable discriminations are being emphasized;

yet I feel that many of us are unnecessarily alarmed at the emergence of the new epoch in the church, and I feel confident that some in their thinking have not done justice to the new point of view underlying the present movement.

The unique possibilities of psychotherapy in its various features are being appreciated at our great medical center in Baltimore, the Johns Hopkins University. Mr. Phipps has just given more than a million dollars for a new department and equipment to study mental diseases, especially in the lines of psychiatry, and many of the leading professors, such as Dr. William H. Welch, Dr. Lewellys F. Barker, Dr. W. S. Thayer, and Dr. Henry M. Hurd, are physicians of most hospitable spirit. It was the sympathy and encouragement of such physicians, especially Dr. Barker and Dr. Hurd, that led me to accept the invitation of the students to deliver the course of addresses given in this volume.

It is a significant sign of the times that a minister should be invited to do this work, but it was accepted as an opportunity for talking over a most vital matter with a choice section of a coming generation of physicians, and feeling the pulse of the future. As the genial physician, Dr. Oliver Wendell Holmes, loved to talk theology with young theologues, so a modern minister may find prophecy and potency in talking vital medicine with the coming neurologists of this wonderful unfolding century.

The new movement of co-operation between physicians and ministers does not mean a practice of medicine by the clergyman, as some contend, but a teaching and practicing of the fundamental principles of mental control and rational living. It does not mean abandoning the ministerial profession, but a new infusion of interest in the vital and practical work of the ministry, and a new realization of the wonderful intimacies of spiritual and physical work.

The real spirit of the new movement is not an attempt to turn clergymen into physicians through a magic use of psychic forces, but it is to make ministers more intelligent and efficient in their God-given ministry of teaching and consolation and also to make them more wisely co-operative with the physicians who share in the care of the sick of their parishes.

We all recognize the perils and the limitations of the movement toward co-operation between physicians and ministers. There are the dangers, as Dr. Cabot puts it, "of seeking help in the wrong place." But co-operation will usually remedy this. There is danger that the "movement may spread too far and too fast." There is, however, too much hard work in it, for it to go very fast. That danger may be taken for granted as righting itself in the long run. There is the danger of "inadequate training." This is true. But it is as true for the physicians as the clergymen. Many physicians are sadly inadequate for their work, and especially for the larger work of psychotherapy. But the work itself sifts out its workers. More than study and training are needed to be effective. It needs fine aptitudes in an understanding both of psychotherapy and of human nature. The movement will gradually correct any extravagancies and find its equilibrium.

The Emmanuel Movement has been an interesting development. It has done great good. It has called attention to some forgotten facts. But it is a question whether its continuance or further extension on its present lines would be wise. For a full discussion of its work from a psychologist's standpoint, and especially its perils from the employment of hypnotism, the reader is referred to a series of three articles in three recent issues of *The Psychological Clinic* by the editor, Dr. Lightner Witmer. These articles are a careful examination, analysis and criticism of the movement, and deserve thoughtful consideration. They commend the social work and the religious appeal of the work, but show its very grave dangers. These present addresses aim to avoid these dangers by excluding the use of hypnotism, and by showing the limitations of the work, as well as by emphasizing the practical side of the work within these limited lines.

It might be a serious calamity to the churches to endeavor to repeat in other parishes that unique experience of the Emmanuel Movement. But I do know from experience how helpfully and practically the essential principles of rational psychotherapy can be used in a parish, and without church clinics and without the least attempt at hypnotic therapeutics, with all the teaching in the open, and all the methods, the tested experience of rational living.

The perils are real, but the practical possibilities are greater. For what we must bear in mind, in general, is, that the new movement emphasizes the fact that we can learn to control our feelings and functions. "A large proportion of nervous patients," Dr. Lewellys F. Barker said recently, in one of his addresses, "are victims of unhealthy emotional states. Instead of being invigorated by healthy feelings, they are exhausted by depression, irritability, worry, fear." They may "learn how to school their emotions," is his hopeful verdict, and "how to cast worry and anger out of their lives. One of the best means of doing this is by encouraging the cultivation in a positive way of the elevating and strengthening emotions and sentiments—appreciation, faith, hope, love and joy. All sham emotions, accompanied by tension and strain, should be banished, and the patient should be taught not to cherish emotion for its own sake, but always to endeavor to give expression to it by the performance of an act with which it accords."

We must remember that the new co-operation really began with the physicians. Dr. Weir Mitchell was the inspiration. A great debt is due also to Dr. Paul DuBois, to Dr. Morton Prince, Dr. J. J. Putman, and many others for their splendid services in the sane and scientific progress of the movement and in showing its limitations. For the future, we believe the largest responsibility and development of the work must be in the physician's hands, the minister's part, when required, being merely co-operative, but nevertheless important.

Some have contended that the primary duty of the church is to the well. The Master did not so discriminate. He acted as if the primary duty were to all the needy, both sick and well. Frequently his first ministrations were to the sick. The clergyman has duties to the well, but also special duties to his sick, a large number in every parish, taking a great deal of his time and strength. He must visit them nearly as often as the doctor,—the duty is enjoined both by the commands of religion and of humanity. How can he most effectively use his visits and opportunities of helping? Surely not in simply talking religion and by praying, but by talking religion and by prayer to some definite purpose; not against physiology and psychology, but in harmony with these; not at cross purposes with the medical man in attendance, but in active and complete co-operation with him. There ought to be a real understanding in this work between the physician and the minister.

One critic advises the minister to let religiously alone this work for which he is unfit. Yes, but in some cases he may be exactly the very one to co-operate with a physician who feels himself unfit for the spiritual factors perchance involved in the case. The pastor can often consult with the physician, even in the diagnosis, and sometimes throw great light on the case by giving certain mental and spiritual factors involved.

Besides, a minister is often the very one who can best give a needed stimulus toward faith, right directions for prayer and a re-education in mental and spiritual outlook. As Dr. Richard Cabot, a wise and conservative Boston physician, says: "Education is indeed the most potent of all our weapons in the attack upon nervous disorders. But it is not academic nor intellectual acumen that we wish to produce in this type of sufferer, but rather that moral and spiritual awakening which gives him a greater and better reason, a purer and intenser motive, for all that he does. Because I believe, then, that all explanation, all encouragement, all education, which ignores religion is for that reason slip-shod and slovenly, I believe that patients whose physical ills can be mitigated through explanation, encouragement and education, need the help of some one to whom religion is a working reality."

Religion as a working reality has therefore its place in the new therapeutics, and I feel that we must recognize that something of permanent value has come,—a new outlook for the minister in his pulpit and pastoral work, and a new possibility of intelligent co-operation between the minister and physician. The minister in this is not practicing medicine. He is merely doing his part toward the health, wholesomeness and holiness of the community. I contend that too much conservatism in this matter is as perilous as an unwise radicalism. We need a large hospitality to new truth and new methods. We need balance, but also faith in the fuller work of the ministry. It is most important in all this new development of possibilities to keep a level head, but keeping a level head does not necessarily mean utterly ignoring providential leadings and leaving religiously alone great fields of moral usefulness and spiritual regeneration that are involved in these new possibilities of mental control and will-power.

I firmly believe that a study of psychotherapy is as important to the modern minister as a study of psychology or sociology. It is really a new adjunct in practical theology. For a fuller exposition of this general point of view, the reader is referred to a very sensible and suggestive series of articles on "Psychotherapy and the Church" which recently appeared in *The Congregationalist* of Boston, by Rev. Chauncey J. Hawkins, which shows, from a clerical standpoint and after a careful study of European clinics, how the psychotherapeutic work in general is best done without connection with religious institutions and yet at the same time how co-operation may be most helpful and how certain phases of the work may enrich and enlarge pastoral service.

Allow me, in a few words, to recapitulate the purpose of this volume. Whatever is worth while in the Christian Science movement, but without its extravagancies and inconsistencies, we want to show in its right relations in these addresses. Whatever is best and wisest in the Emmanuel Movement, but without its clinics and hypnotic treatments, we want clearly and strongly to emphasize.

We aim to set forth the essentials of a wise co-operation between physicians and ministers in their mutual care of the sick; but just as clearly we aim to show the methods of self-treatment along these efficacious lines of mental and spiritual control. In a word, we aim at something of permanent value, independent of all passing movements, in the themes that we shall consider.

These addresses are for the well as emphatically as for the sick. They aim at prevention as well as cure. Our point of view is rational psychotherapy, with the addition, when needed, of spiritual suggestion and the re-education of the whole mental outlook toward God and man.

The special studies that I have been following in these lines for the past ten years, I am sure, have enriched my own ministry, both in sermonic directness and appeal, and in practical helpfulness in pastoral visitations. These conclusions are not hasty ones. Nine years ago, in a published pamphlet of lectures before the University of Maryland and church conferences, and some time earlier than the Emmanuel Movement was conceived, I contended that "the basis that is really vital in Christian Science teaching, without its extravagancies and inconsistencies,—we have been preaching and practicing in this church of ours for years, and the same might be said of many another church in this city. This is what we mean. We have been preaching cheerfulness, optimism, don't worry, calmness. We have been preaching faith in God and the healing power of God's love in the whole life. We have been preaching the supremacy of the spirit, that nothing is eternal but the soul and God. We have been constantly trying to make our church an assembly of hopeful, healthy minds, and by that means to re-inforce every physician's work and to give to every heart the uplifting realization of the very presence of God. As a matter of fact, this very church of ours, to use a further concrete illustration, although the same statement might truly be made of many another church in this city—this very church of ours is a greater curative agency than any Christian Science church in Baltimore or Boston. We have seven or more excellent physicians as members of our congregation. The pastor by his preaching and in his pastoral visitation, counsel and prayers, as well as in more direct ways, aims to co-operate with every one of these in healing processes. The pastor's prayers and preaching and visiting are all in the line of the awakening of faith and the promoting of cheerfulness and the emphasizing of the good promises and good purposes of God. The pastor and these seven physicians have not taken written testimonials during the past year, nor have they talked about them, and yet we are well assured that there are hundreds of cases of cures, positive cures, wrought this past year by the co-operating agencies of this church. We have used good nursing, some medicine when necessary, and a strong infusion of reasonableness and Christian faith. We have not despised medicine, wisely given to assist nature, for we have obtained through medicine a far larger percentage of cures than the Christian Scientists without medicine. We can reach more cases. As a matter of fact, the Christian Scientists have nothing but what we have and can use, and besides faith and hope and will-power which we instill, we also use the best skill and experience of trained physicians. Indeed, as a matter of plain fact, so far the very best institution of real Christian Science, of genuine healing power, in this city is the Johns Hopkins Hospital,—a noble outcome of both true Christianity and true science."

OLIVER HUCKEL.

BALTIMORE, April 10, 1909.

INTRODUCTION

DURING the past winter the Rev. Dr. Oliver Huckel acceded to the request of the Young Men's Christian Association of the Johns Hopkins Medical School to give a series of talks upon the methods of helping troubled minds which had proven useful to him in his pastoral experience. These talks were highly valued by the students who were privileged to listen to them; and now that Dr. Huckel has consented to publish them, they will, I feel sure, discover a large circle of appreciative readers.

Medical men and clergymen do not always agree regarding fundamental principles, but as medicine becomes more enlightened and religion more liberal, there is an ever widening area of common ground on which the representatives of these two great professions may meet and co-operate. Though there has been strife between religion and science, there is no conflict between medical truth and religious truth; where there is contention we may be sure that on one side or the other, or on both sides, the truth is only partially revealed.

A field which has always been of interest, both to the physician and the clergyman, is that of the milder mental disturbances to which a large contingent of the human race is subject. It falls to the lot of every pastoral worker to comfort the troubled and depressed, to soothe the disturbed, to try to stimulate the apathetic, to attempt to quiet the unduly exalted, to help to strengthen the enfeebled will, to chide the faulty and negligent, and to rebuke the morally delinquent and depraved. It is a part of the work of medical men to recognize and treat anomalies of the intellect, the emotions and the will; to deal with disturbances of sensation, of memory, of attention, of feeling, of judgment, of voluntary motion or conduct and of the involuntary motor activities which are known as reflexes and instincts. Clergymen deal with these matters in their own way, and physicians, independently, have worked out their special methods for managing them. For a long time it seemed scarcely to be recognized that clergymen and physicians were trying to solve similar, if not in many instances identical, problems, but recently the recognition has become more general. Considering the progress of the doctrine of psycho-physical parallelism this is by no means surprising; it is strange only that people should regard it as strange.

There can be but little doubt that all work as yet in the field of mental medicine is to be looked upon as rudimentary, but the application of the exact methods of psychologists, studying normal mental processes, and of psychiatrists, analyzing diseased mental states, is gradually supplying the data for a foundation upon which a sound mental medicine may be built up.

It has often occurred to me that physicians are prone to be so interested in the physical side of their patients that they sometimes neglect the study of the psychic state, and I have also, for a long time, felt that clergymen are inclined, on account of their interest in the moral and spiritual side of man, to lose sight of the physical and to hold men responsible for and to condemn as "sinful," acts and mental attitudes which are the determined activities of disordered brains.

There are some medical men who believe that it is a mistake for clergymen to make any effort to help the disordered mind, maintaining that all such "cases" belong to the physician. On the other hand there would appear to be some clergymen who regard the inquiries of a medical man who resorts to modern methods of psycho-analysis as an infringement upon the prerogatives of a profession, whose work it is to deal with the affairs of the human "soul." Both these attitudes seem to me unfair and illogical. though I am ready to grant that there is danger of grave mistakes being made by both groups of workers.

It seems to me, therefore, all the more desirable that the minister should understand the attitude of physicians, and that the medical man should try to learn the point of view of the clergyman. Let each give of his best to the other and let each welcome warnings of feet that go astray!

LEWELLYS F. BARKER.

BALTIMORE, April 6, 1909.

FIRST CONFERENCE

Mental and Spiritual Factors in the Problem of Health

I. The New Outlook For Health.
II. The Unique Powers of the Mind.
III. The Spiritual Mastery of the Body.

I. THE NEW OUTLOOK FOR HEALTH

DO you remember Thomas Carlyle's ideal of health, notable from one who had wretched health most of his life, a desperate digestion and consequently a savage temper. Nevertheless he had an ideal of health, and it was this: "In the midst of your zeal and ardor remember the care of health. . . . It would have been a very great thing for me if I had been able to consider that health is a thing to be attended to continually, that you are to regard good health as the very highest of all temporal things for you. There is no kind of achievement you can make in the world that is equal to perfect health. What to it are nuggets and millions? The French financier said, 'Why is there no sleep to be sold!' Sleep was not in the market at any quotation." He continues: "You could not get any better definition of what 'holy' really is than 'healthy.' Completely healthy means, 'mens sana in corpore sano.' a man all lucid and in equilibrium. His intellect a clear mirror, brilliantly sensitive to all objects and impressions made on it, and showing all things in their correct proportions; healthy, clear and free." That was Carlyle's vision of perfect health.

We are now in the days of specialists, and a most necessary and admirable work they are doing. But even the specialization of functions has its limitations and its inadequacies. For a "man is not made up in air-tight compartments, each of which can be treated as an entirety, wholly separable from the rest of his life," nor is man merely "a bundle of organs, each of which can be safely handed over to a specialist, and health thereby secured." There is coming to be a new insistence in these days on the close and intimate relationship of all parts of the body and the subtle sympathy in health or disease that pervades the whole system. In other words, greater recognition is being given to the integer man,—the whole man, a living organism in one undivided totality from center to circumference, through soul, and mind and body. And therefore, it is being realized that in many cases of medical treatment, not merely one organ but the whole man must be taken into consideration and treated.

The age of specialists has also brought into prominence, as perhaps never before, the alarming evidence that the prevailing maladies of our day are nervous and functional disorders. These are the facts, as given in various medical authorities. A large part of the diseases of modern times are entirely mental, so-called imaginary, various forms of hypochondria. A large part are mentally induced. A large part are of the protean malady of our age,—nervous troubles,—which are largely mental and partly physical. And only a comparatively small percentage are simply and entirely physical.

Therefore, a science which studies only the workings of material factors upon a material organization may be well enough as far as it goes, but it is not fully adequate for the prevailing and desperate needs of our day. Mind plays a large part in every phase and action of bodily life. Mental factors must be more largely recognized and taken into account. Medical schools have been slow in doing this work. In consequence, there has grown up in our day various so-called curative agencies which seek to supplement the medical profession. They are mostly irregular systems, many of them illogical and entirely unscientific, some of them full of absurdities and charlatanism. Yet we are being taught in these days, even by these movements in more distinct ways than ever, the wonderful influence of mind over matter, of brain over body.

It is acknowledged that the greatest field for mental medicine is co-operation with physical treatment in the restoration of the nerves to equilibrium, right adjustment and normal action. The disorders of the nervous system are the most numerous class of ailments in our day. The nervous system itself is most complex and of infinite delicacy. Its diseases are subtle and diffused in the system, often affecting separate parts, or the whole system. Its symptoms are most varied, the classification of its forms most difficult.

It was formerly customary to speak of the general condition as nervous prostration. Now it is usually referred to as neurasthenia. But neurasthenia has many special forms and varieties, each with its separate scientific name. We need not go into the classification or description; you know well enough in general what they are.

"What is ordinarily called nervousness," says one writer, "is not a disease, but a condition, the result of overstrain or overstimulation of the nervous system. The most healthy person may feel this at times. But it may pass off through rest or better conditions. But when it becomes acute and long continued, and causes general physical debility, then it has become a disease and is called neurasthenia."

According to Dr. William Osler, the three great advances of the century made by the medical profession have been a knowledge of the mode of controlling epidemic diseases, the introduction of anæsthetics, and the adoption of antiseptic methods in surgery.

"Think," he says, "of the Nemesis which has overtaken pain during the past fifty years. Anæsthetics and antiseptic surgery have almost manacled the demon, and since their introduction the aggregate of pain which has been prevented far outweighs in civilized communities that which has been suffered."

He says again: "The sorrows and troubles of men, it is true, have not been materially diminished, but bodily pain and suffering, though not abolished, have been assuaged as never before, and the share of each in the 'weltschmerz' had been enormously lessened."

Now while it is true that tuberculosis, diphtheria, yellow fever, and the whole brood of contagious and infectious diseases have been yielding to the attack of medical science and steadily diminishing, nervous disorders have been increasing at an alarming rate, and it is recognized that new medical factors must be brought forward to meet this crisis. Therefore, psychotherapy is being studied as one most promising factor in the problem. As one says:

"A courageous, hopeful attitude of mind, even though indirectly, helps in the fight against most diseases. But in functional nervous disorders, which have an origin largely mental, thoughts and ideas can be made direct remedies." John Hunter, a noted surgeon and a most scientific and practical-minded man, once said, "As one state of mind is capable of producing disease, another state of mind effects the cure."

Dr. Paul DuBois of Berne maintains that nervousness is often a disease pre-eminently psychic, and a psychic disease needs psychic treatment. Then he asks this question: "Can we by means of the mind often escape illness, prevent functional troubles, diminish or suppress those which already exist?" And in his opinion, backed by long experience, this is certainly possible.

"The care of the human being as a whole soul and body, is increasingly coming to the front," says Dr. A. T. Schofield. And in the same way the wise physician must grasp the underlying unity of the spiritual and the material, and recognize that if the body may and does influence the diseases of the soul, so does the mind influence states and diseases of the body. "I utterly refuse," he continues, "to regard the mental factor in medicine as a retrogression. It is, on the contrary, a step, and a great step, in advance, for the day is past when the physician can limit his knowledge and practice to the physical." *

Professor Ladd, in an article in the *Medical Times,* says: "The effects capable of being produced by mind on body are very clear, real and considerable, and while in all ages they have been the chief therapeutic

* Dr. Schofield—*The Mental Factor in Medicine.*

agents on which the charlatan and quack have relied, they have probably been less trusted and utilized by the scientific physician than experience warrants or psychology suggests."

Dr. Charles K. Mills, professor of neurology at the University of Pennsylvania, has called attention to this distinction in an article on "Psychotherapy: its Scope and Limitations."* He says: "Psychic medicine and mystic medicine are terms sometimes used as if they were interchangeable. This is not the exact truth. In a certain sense mystic medicine is psychic medicine, but the reverse does not, or at least should not, hold good. In the incantations of the medicine men, of the savages, in the appeals to omens and to oracles, in the calling upon the sun and the stars to relieve the sick and the helpless, in the ministrations of Mrs. Eddy and her apostles, in the resort to healing shrines of every description, the psychic element is easily discoverable. These and other forms of mystic healing appeal to the superstition or the imagination of the individual; they play both upon his normal and abnormal suggestibility.

* Monthly Cyclopedia and Medical Bulletin, July 1908.)

They do this, however, not from the standpoint of the sane and scientific believer in the proper use of suggestion. They attribute cures to supernatural interferences, and in this way deceive in the very act of helping. The psychic medicine in which the doctor should be continuously interested is that in which the use of mental influences is as the use of water, medicine, electricity, the surgeon's knife, or the forceps of the obstetrician."

The psychotherapy which makes the very least possible use of hypnotism, and which depends largely on methods of absolute sincerity with the patient, and the re-education of the mentality with the conscious co-operation of the patient, is the line of work which is most commending itself to thoughtful people in these days. As Dr. Charles K. Mills continues: "DuBois comes to us saying that the best psychotherapeutic method is that of reasoning or persuasion, that of informing the patient as to the nature of his case and of reasoning him into the belief that it is curable, and that he (the patient) can help out this cure. This is not a new plan of curing or attempting to cure the sick. It has existed wherever good physicians have used their mental powers for their fellows. The doctor of the metropolis, of the town or of the cross-roads, if one well fitted for his vocation, has successfully exercised this art of persuasion, as he has also that of appealing to blind faith. A debt however is due to DuBois, to Prince, to Putman, and to others working in this field, for concentrating the attention of the profession on the value of persuasive or reasoning methods, and on the best way of using them for the relief of nervous ills. Methods of education and of persuasion have been illuminated by them and, in so far as such methods are more clearly seen and better understood, are likely to be more largely and effectively employed." Suggestion probably enters into all psychotherapy, but in the educational method is more than mere suggestion.

So also, Dr. Richard M. Cabot gives testimony: "Let us bear in mind that it is by a catholic inclusiveness of all that is good in many methods of attacking disease, and by an effective combination of explanation, education, command (or suggestion) joined with all the other therapeutic resources, psychic, chemical, and physical, that the American type of psychotherapeutics can hope for success. Let us search for no panacea, neglect no aspect of human nature, make no exclusive appeal to the conscious, the subconscious, the physical, chemical or biological sides of human nature. We want to cure the whole man, not any section of him. Is it not obvious, then, that we should study every element of human nature, and try to understand as best we may the complex interactions and team work of body and soul?"

It is an earnest company of eminent scientific men who have been working to put the whole subject of psychotherapeutics on a rational basis. Prominent among them are, Liebault, Bernheim, Janet, Forel, DuBois, Moll, Meyers, Braid, Bramewell, Oppenheim, Schofield; and in our own country, William James, Mark Baldwin, Morton Prince, Lewellys F. Barker, W. J. Hudson, Isador H. Coriat, James J. Putman, Frederick Peterson, Boris Sidis, Wood, Dresser, and a hundred more. The careful and unique explorations of these scientific investigators into the subconsciousness of patients suffering with various nervous disorders have given results most interesting and important and have revealed marvelous possibilities of the human mind.

Some of these men are doing inestimable service, especially in disclosing the subconscious and subliminal realms. Others through their "fresh, strong, inspirational thinking, are doing valiant pioneering upon both the spiritual and human sides of the heretofore great divide," and are elucidating deep things in their new thinking, while others along more technical lines are turning "psychologic knowledge into therapeutic account," and are calling upon the entire medical profession to see and be convinced of the power of mind in many cases to cure many bodily diseases.

Now what possible part has religion in this work?

As to the direct helpfulness of a minister's work in co-operation with physicians, we may look at the large and broad value of the Christian spirit and truth.. Dr. Matthews states in his recommendation of right thinking as necessary to right acts and results: "Christianity is the greatest teacher of right thinking, and its wonderful power to prevent disease is just beginning to be realized. That it is the greatest power in the world to prevent disease no doctor who has had practice and experience enough to know doubts. No one can realize better than a doctor what an amazingly large percentage of diseases result from immorality, dissipation, and weak will-power, from ignorance, from unclean thinking and unclean living—in short from leading lives the Bible condemns on every page. Perhaps fifty per cent. of all diseases is due directly or indirectly to these causes. Can Christianity prevent fifty per cent. of the sickness that now prevails? I believe it can. But it must be directed to that end. Electricity is a great power. Applied one way it produces heat; in another way, light; in another it moves machinery; in another it transmits messages. So Christianity applied in one way civilizes and lifts up; in another way it purifies the heart; in another it prevents disease. There will be a great awakening throughout the world when people realize that Christianity prevents disease and adds years to human life. It pays to be a Christian right here in this world, without any reference to a future world."

Such helpful teaching, concerning the fundamentals of normal and wholesome living can be given from the pulpit and in pastoral visiting, and in personal relations with the people.

Still another way in which the minister can help is by special courses of health-sermons from time to time in his church. These may be made to supplement the general teaching of Christianity by definite applications to the problems of health. There is a real gospel of the body. Such a general line of thought and teaching as is indicated in the themes of these addresses might be sufficient for these teachings. It might also be wise to have health classes for yet fuller study along these lines, but it is a doubtful experiment to inaugurate church-clinics for the cure of disease. This work had much better be left to the regular physicians.

Besides this, however, a minister, if he is wise and interested in these things, may often co-operate most helpfully with a physician in regard to certain cases, giving his aid at the request of the physician under his direction. There are nervous diseases which need emphatically the fullest help in physical, mental and spiritual ways. The minister can often furnish the spiritual factor that is needed, and be of real service.

There is still another more direct method of co-operation and helpfulness. The pastor can often consult with the physician, even in the diagnosis, and sometimes throw great light on the case by giving the mental or spiritual factors involved. A patient will frequently tell his pastor certain things that he would not think to mention to a medical man, and yet these items may mean a great deal in understanding the patient's real history and condition and the definite needs and treatment.

As Dr. MacDonald has also borne testimony: "Often the first help of cure is 'confession,' wherein the patient unburdens himself of his worries, confesses his follies and indulgences that go back for years, perhaps, holding him in chains and binding him to his present diseased condition. There is large benefit to the sufferer in this opportunity to free his mind to a sympathetic listener. It also opens avenues for insight into the nature of a person's malady, so that curative suggestion can be the easier applied. We all know the value of a heart-to-heart talk with one who can enter into our grief sympathetically. It relaxes and rests us. The old restrictions become unloosed. We experience a sense of freedom and ease. And if the person to whom we confide the secret of our discontent has the ability to help us out of our misery, our very confidence in him has curative force." *

Closely allied to this is the so-called psycho-analysis, one of the newer psychological methods of discovering the mental conditions causing nervous disorders. This method, as one describes it, is a "kind of detective which turns the subconsciousness inside out like a glove and brings to light hidden causes of nervous trouble, a shock, perhaps, emotional or physical, a grief, a fancied injury, which the patient sometimes has forgotten entirely but which, hidden in the depths of consciousness, has been working like a poison. Akin to this is the intimate talk we have with those who come as patients which reveals a life's experience and gives the understanding of temperament necessary for an intelligent handling of the case. In these conversations disclosures are made of suffering in the inner life of thought and feeling that has never been confessed to the nearest and dearest of friends and relatives. . . . Each case is a law unto itself and the cause that often underlies the apparent cause must be discov-

* Robert MacDonald—*Mind, Religion and Health.*

ered and overcome before a wholesome condition of mind can be established." *

But in all this personal relation with the sick, both ministers and physicians must be perfectly frank and honest with patients,—no deception or subterfuges. We must have their absolute confidence and trust in order to do them good. No deception about present conditions and no false promises for the future. But this does not mean that we should exaggerate conditions. It is just as bad to be an alarmist. It is false treatment to look on the dark side. If there is a single ray of hope, any scintilla of light, then it is the physician's bounden duty, or the minister's, if he have the physician's consent, to give encouragement, to suggest hope and courage, to make continually what Dr. Cabot calls "creative assertions."

In a word, in psychotherapy, either purely mental, or mental and spiritual combined, the object is not merely to give a few specific ideas and directions, but also to create an atmosphere in which these ideas may work. The object of these addresses is, both to give the great essential ideas that inspire new life, new hope, new health, and also to create at

* Fallows—*Health and Happiness.*

the same time the right atmosphere in the mind and spirit, so that the ideals will have a good soil in which to grow. This is not done in a single half hour, but requires longer periods of time.

When we talk about health, we mean both spiritual and bodily health. We are emphasizing a neglected truth when we are asserting that the laws of health are the laws of God, and that sin and sickness are very intimately associated in God's universe. The true gospel does not really begin with its outward treatments, but it seeks instantly to get a hold on the soul. It begins with the sources of life. It is, therefore, not merely a system of therapeutics, but a religion that seeks to be therapeutic.

This is the idea in a nutshell, as Rev. Charles A. Place puts it: "The first step is to free a man from the idea that he is a victim of some strange power by showing him the real cause; then the demand is to build up his moral control and confidence in himself. To accomplish this latter, the soul must be awakened to the worth of its own powers and how to use them and led out of all narrowness to a richer life with man and with God. This is the all-important work of the minister, dealing directly with the soul and its sources of strength within and without, and combining sound psychology and sound religion."

Personally, I believe that the full direction of this new movement must ultimately rest with the physicians, and that the ministers, if they remain in it at all, shall merely aid in special ways under the supervision and cordial consent of the physicians. Conservative and scientific methods must be used even in advance work. Special courses in colleges and medical schools will doubtless be instituted for the purpose of rendering more efficient service. The preliminary diagnosis and psychic analysis will gradually become more definite and illuminating and we may "reasonably expect that the satisfactory results will be proportionately larger."

We must, however, recognize the fact that this age in which we live is characterized by a new hope and a new outlook for health. Such great truths as these are coming to the front. God wills health for us. It is not God's wish or will that any one of us shall suffer. He wants us well,—physically, spiritually well—every whit whole. He wants us normal and perfect. That is God's idea for us. It is, therefore, both foolish and wicked to endure ill-health and disease so long as there is any hope or means of cure.

Another truth is coming to the fore: All's law,—but all's love. All is law,—God's law, both natural and spiritual. And it is the invariability and reliability of all God's law that is their kindness.

The laws of health are God's laws,—both natural and spiritual. Obeyed, they bring health; broken, they bring sickness. There is God's kindness and love in this law of consequences.

In the ordinary civil life, if we flagrantly break the law, we are punished. Ignorance of the law does not excuse us. It is our business to learn the law and keep it. So in the matter of health; ignorance of the laws of health will not excuse us. We must learn the law and keep it. All our sickness comes to us either by our ignorance or our wilfulness or through ignorance or wilfulness of others,—ancestors, parents, nurses or friends.

This truth is gaining wider acceptance. God never arbitrarily sends sickness upon us as punishment, test or discipline, but it comes always as a penalty for broken laws, broken consciously or unconsciously, broken by ourselves or by our ancestors, or by others who influence us.

We must learn God's laws and obey them. We cannot dissipate and expect good health; the law will exact its penalties; we cannot be gluttons in eating and expect good health; we cannot burn the candle at both ends and expect steady nerves. Back of every physical ailment, there is a broken law. We must learn God's laws and obey them.

A further truth is that we cannot *demand* health from God; we must follow God's laws. We need not *pray* for health,—it will be useless—unless we are willing to fulfil the conditions. Our whole purpose must be to learn the fundamental laws of God for health, for they are all harmonious, and then to put the divine principles into daily practice.

But how far do we know the laws of health? How far may we learn these fundamental principles of well-being? We cannot say that we know them all,—there are still mysteries and undiscovered laws. But we already know enough to help us all toward better living and into better health. We already know more than we practice.

But someone asks,—How are we transgressing God's law, when walking along the street we are caught by some disease germs in the air from a passing stranger and become sick? We are not, of course, consciously transgressing, but we are transgressing God's laws unless we keep ourselves in such good condition that we can resist germs. Germs take hold of weak, run-down physical condition. Here is where the transgression is manifest. We have no right to let ourselves run down physically; it is our duty to keep in prime condition. Then we are practically immune.

But what of epidemics of small-pox or yellow-fever? How does transgression come in where the plague seems to attack everybody indiscriminately, even those in good condition? It is, indeed, perplexing; but we may say: Often an epidemic comes because of transgression, not of an individual, but of a community or city, in not providing sanitary conditions, or in not taking the rightful sanitary precautions.

Even in such conditions as these, mental and spiritual matters count. For instance, those who are not afraid are usually immune. If we get rid of fear we are far less liable to attack. It is fear that weakens and kills.

Another truth is receiving new emphasis.

Pain is not a penalty, punishment or discipline,—not something merely disagreeable that has to be endured. It is a danger signal to tell us we are doing wrong—that something is deranged in our life. We must not go on but stop and see what is wrong, and right it. Pain is like the notice often put up at railroad crossings: "Stop, look, listen!" See what is wrong; right it if you are able; retrieve the broken law. Pain, therefore, is a friendly adviser, a kindly friend, a messenger from God. God sends pain in this sense, never arbitrarily, but to teach us His laws and how to obey them.

Now all these truths are important because we want to create in souls the spirit of resistance to disease and diseased moods and habits, and a determination to fight against sickness with all the means that God puts into our hands. We want to get rid of the acquiescent and passive mood in the presence of disease. We must realize that we are in this fight in accordance with God's will. We must remember that He approves of our effort and fight for health; and we must be sure,—for it is a fact,—that He will assist us in this fight for health in every possible way. We are made for health; we are made for happiness; and the life that attains nearest to both these things is usually the life that has come into fullest harmony with God. Harmony, then, is what we teach and preach,—harmony with God's laws, harmony with God's will. For it is not physical health alone that is the object of life, but the health of the spirit, the health of the whole life.

Many people in these days are spoiling their lives for lack of knowledge or lack of care in these fundamentals of rational living and good health. We want to remind them of certain great facts and principles which they ought to know, or if they do know, have forgotten how to use.

We believe that the church has a great duty and service that it can render in putting the emphasis more strenuously on these things that make for right living. It has worked somewhat along these lines all through the centuries. We believe that it can do this work yet more systematically and effectively. It must get away from morbid teachings, morbid emotions and morbid moods in religion. It must emphasize the wholesome and optimistic heart of true religion.

May we remind you again that these are not medical lectures, but spiritual addresses. We shall aim to consider health through the inner springs of life, through the divine and latent forces in the life, through the re-education of the man in the first principles of right living. We shall aim to help methods of healing by an appeal to the regulative and recuperative faculties of the mind, when stimulated and strengthened by a new infusion of faith and prayer. We shall aim to show that the essential principles of religion are in fullest harmony with the latest findings of science, as revealed in psychology and physiology.

We must not, however, expect impossibilities. Only a certain class of cases can be met and helped in this way. Other cases, where the trouble is exceptional, or where the cause is organic derangement, must seek the advice and treatment of the best physicians. But many cases, we are sure, need only mental stimulus and spiritual outlook.

In the care of our bodies we must not neglect our souls. We must save both body and soul. We work for the redemption of the entire life.

II. THE UNIQUE POWERS OF MIND

CONSIDER the unique influence of mind over body. We are recognizing it as a singular and marvelous power. It has been manifested in all ages. It has been studied carefully and systematically only in the last few generations.

May I recall to you two or three instances that show very strikingly the power of mind over body?

Take such an incident as this, which is related by General Grant in his Memoirs: "The night before General Lee's surrender General Grant was suffering so acutely from a headache that he could not sleep. It was a splitting headache and no wonder, with the gallant Lee to contend with. He spent the night trying vainly to alleviate the pain; bathing his feet in hot water and mustard, and putting hot mustard plasters on his wrists and on the back part of his neck. When the officer bearing General Lee's letter reached him, he writes: 'I was still suffering from the sick headache, but the instant I saw the contents of the note, I was cured.' "

It is related that "during the naval fight off Santiago, while the *Oregon* was pushing after the *Cristobal Colon*, under forced draught, the stokers were nearly overcome by their great labor, and the tremendous heat of the hold. As yet she had not partaken in the fight. The chief engineer, noticing the condition of his men, signaled up to Captain Clark, 'Give them a gun.' The gun was given—and exhaustion passed away in the excitement of the belief that the battle had begun."

Hundreds of similar cases might be cited. This incident is well authenticated: Once at Weimar, Luther found Melancthan very ill. His eyes were dim, his tongue faltering, his understanding almost gone. "Alas," complained Luther, "that the devil should have thus unstrung so fine an instrument." Then he knelt beside his sick friend and prayed. Soon he stood up and cried, "Be of good cheer, Philip; you shall not die. It is God's delight to impart life, not to inflict death. Trust in the Lord for He can impart new life." And Melancthan recovered from his illness.

It is related that when Benvenuto Cellini was about to cast his famous statue of Perseus, now in the Loggia dei Lanzi at Florence, he was taken with a sudden fever and forced to go home to bed. In the midst of his suffering, one of his workmen rushed in to say: "O Benvenuto, your statue is spoiled, and there is no hope whatever of saving it." Dressing hastily, he rushed to his furnace and found his metal "caked." Ordering dry oak wood brought in, he fired the furnace fiercely, working in a rain that was falling, stirred the channels, and saved his metal. He continues the story thus: "After all was over, I turned to a plate of salad on a bench there and ate with a hearty appetite, and drank together with the whole crew. Afterward I retired to my bed, healthy and happy, for it was now two hours before morning, and slept as sweetly as though I had never felt a touch of illness." His overpowering idea of saving his statue drove away the physical condition and left him well.

Someone asked Dr. Elisha Kane, the Arctic explorer, to give the best proved instance that he knew of the soul's power over the body. He paused a moment upon the question, as if to feel how it was put, and answered as with a spring: "The soul can lift the body out of its boots, sir! When our captain was dying—I say dying—I have seen scurvy enough to know—every old scar on his body an ulcer—I never saw a case so bad that either lived or died of it, usually long before they are as ill as he was—there was trouble abroad. There might be mutiny as soon as the breath was out of his body. We might be at each other's throats. I felt that he owed the repose of the dying to the service. I went down to his bunk and shouted in his ear, 'Mutiny, Captain, mutiny!' He shook off the cadaverous stupor. 'Set me up!' said he, 'and order these fellows before me!' He heard the complaint, ordered punishment, and from that hour convalesced."

It is stated that scientific experiments by Prof. W. G. Anderson of Yale University, recently, succeeded in practically weighing the result of thought's action. A student was poised on a balance so that the center of gravity of his body was exactly over its center. Set to solving mathematical problems, the increased weight of blood at his head, during the process of calculation, changed his center of gravity and caused an immediate dip of the balance to that side. Repeating the nine multiplication table caused a greater displacement than repeating the table of fives, and in general, the displacement grew greater with greater intensity of thought. Carrying the experiment further, the experimenter had the student imagine himself going through leg gymnastics. As he performed the feats mentally, one by one, the blood flowed to the limbs in quantities sufficient to tip the balance according to the movement thought ,of. By purely mental action the center of gravity of the body was shifted four inches, or as much as by raising the doubled arms over the shoulders. These experiments were repeated on a large number of students with the same results. *

Now, if mind has such influence over body, as seems to be indicated in these instances, is it not reasonable to suppose that mental action can also do much in the control of the nerves and nervous disorders? It has been clearly demonstrated that mental power has such control, and can be most effectively used.

As Hudson says: "No scientist will deny

* Noted by Dr. Marden in *Every Man a King.*

the existence within us of a central intelligence which controls the bodily functions, and through the sympathetic nervous system actuates the involuntary muscles and keeps the bodily machinery in motion. Nor will the most pronounced materialist deny that this central intelligence is the controlling energy which regulates the action of each of the myriad cellular entities of which the whole body is composed."

There are at least five or six irregular curative agencies in the modern world that claim our attention, so strikingly do they illustrate this power of mind over body. Take, for instance, the cures made by the Indian medicine men. Those who have lived among the Indians as government agents and missionaries have borne testimony that they were astonished to find that what they had regarded as the absolute superstition of the belief in medicine men, was something that seemed to have value; that there were most remarkable cures effected by the dances, croonings and incantations of the medicine men.

Cures made at Roman shrines are well known. All through France and Italy there are these wonder-working images and shrines, and sometimes there are hundreds of votive tablets and offerings left at the shrine by those who have been healed,—gold watches, necklaces, diamonds, crutches, and all sorts of testimonials in metal and marble. The cures at St. Anne du Beaupré, near Quebec, in Canada, have been officially noted and examined and certified to by the French physicians.

Cures through popular superstitions are authenticated. There are many contemporary records that show that the cure of scrofula or King's Evil by the touch of the king was more than superstition. In many cases it really effected cures, as certified to by the London physicians of that day. There are recorded instances of stigmata appearing on the body in five places of the wounds of Christ,—like the famous case of St. Francis of Assisi. Several modern cases, such as the one in a hypnotic subject in a Paris hospital, were cured by persistently changing the thought from the passion of Christ to some other theme.

Numerous cures have been wrought by patent medicines, some of which may be excellent, but most of which are worthless. Yet if the absolutely worthless one is well advertised, it never fails to effect some remarkable cures. No medicine on the market but what has hundreds of splendid testimonials of cures actually wrought in some way by and through that medicine. And, finally, there are constant cures made by non-efficacious remedies in physicians' practice. Physicians at the University of Pennsylvania tell of experiments with wooden magnets which often produced the same results and the same cure as the metal ones. An Edinburgh physician records in his autobiography that some of the most remarkable cures in his life-long service were effected by bread pills.

Dr. Clouston, the eminent Scotch physician, says in his enlightening book on the "Hygiene of the Mind": "Certain diseases of impaired nutrition, from warts up to internal tumors, from scurvy to dropsy, have unquestionably been cured by mental influences. This is perfectly explicable from what we know of the relation of the brain to the blood supply of the body. Through the vaso-motor brain function it can be shut off, or give an extra supply of blood to almost any part of the body if the proper stimulus is applied, and thus cure diseases which are due to excess or too scanty supply of blood to any particular part. Imagination, expectation, faith, joy, hope, fear, suggestion, may cure certain diseases."

The record is given in the *British Foreign Medical Review* of a case reported by a naval surgeon as follows: A very intelligent officer had suffered for years from violent attacks of cramps in the stomach. These attacks came on frequently and sub-nitrate of bismuth had been used with good results, but, notwithstanding that the dose was increased to the largest extent that its poisonous qualities would justify, it lost its effect. He was then told that on the next week he would be put under the effect of a medicine which was generally believed to be almost infallible but which was rarely used because of its dangerous quality, but that notwithstanding these, it would be tried, provided he gave his consent. This he did willingly. Accordingly, on the first attack after this, a powder containing four grains was administered every seven minutes, while the greatest anxiety was expressed (within the hearing of the patient) lest too much should be given. The fourth dose caused an entire cessation of pain. Half drachm doses of bismuth had never produced the same relief in three hours. Four times this remedy was used afterward with the same efficacious results. The curative powder was nothing but ship-biscuit ground very fine. Such a special incident may be accounted for by the unusual stimulus of mental action under the thought of the strong drug being administered.

Now, what in general is indicated by the various instances of well-known facts in the healing of disease through Indian medicine men, Roman shrines, popular superstitions, patent medicines, and various cults of faith-healing and Mrs. Eddy's method? They may be said at least to indicate the wonderful power that mind often has over matter, sometimes in the cause, sometimes in the cure of a disease. All these cure about the some percentage—ten to fifteen per cent.

All these various curative agencies are limited to a certain line of diseases,—chiefly nervous troubles in their various forms, which frequently simulate symptoms of heart trouble or consumption, as well as some functional complaints or irregularities of the circulatory system. Sometimes there are rumors and hearsays of the cure of all diseases under the sun, but it is exceedingly hard to find thoroughly authenticated cases of the cure of anything but nervous or hypochondriac troubles.

One of the most interesting questions in our discussion, however, comes at this point. What is the secret of the psychic cure of disease such as is manifested at times in all of these curative agencies?

Three phases of phenomena seem to lead up to the secret of the whole matter.

1. First, there is the healing power of Nature. It is acknowledged by the medical profession that fully ten per cent. of cases would get well if entirely left alone. Just call in Dr. Diet and Dr. Quiet, and give Nature a chance. It is also acknowledged in nearly all diseases that good nursing is half the battle. Sir John Marshall, of London, said: "The vis medicatrix naturae (the healing, the recuperative power of Nature) is the agent to employ in the healing of an ulcer, in the union of a broken bone; the physician or surgeon only assists the natural processes of cure performed by the inherent conservative energy of the frame." And Dr. John Forbes said, in like manner: "In a large proportion of cases, the disease is cured by Nature and not by the physicians.

In a lesser, but still a large proportion, the disease is cured by Nature in spite of the physicians; in other words, their interference rather retards instead of assisting. And in a considerable proportion of diseases, it would fare as well or better with patients if all remedies,—at least all active remedies, especially drugs,—were abandoned. So it comes about that physicians themselves are using fewer drugs in their practice than formerly, and their chief work is merely to assist Nature, —to make conditions such as to give Nature a chance.

2. Further, in all mere cures, there are the effects of ordinary mind force over bodily functions. This is shown in the ordinary experiences of our daily life. Our mental emotions of fright, for instance, or of worry and anxious solicitude, are registered in the retardation of bodily function.

"Where are you going?" asked an Oriental pilgrim of the Plague one day. "I am going to Bagdad to kill 5,000 people," was the reply. A few weeks later the pilgrim met the Plague returning. "You told me you were going to Bagdad to kill 5,000 people," said he, "but instead you killed 50,000." "No," said the Plague, "I only killed 5,000 as I said I would. The others died of fright."

Dr. Robert Macdonald cites this incident.

A volunteer in the recent Spanish-American war lay sick with typhoid fever in a Southern hospital. The physician passing through the ward on his tour of inspection noticed his weakened condition and said to the nurse in attendance, "That man can't live." The young man overheard the remark, and with what remaining strength he had cried out, "I will live!" The physician's remark aroused his antagonism and impelled an auto-suggestion contradictory to the physician's declaration. The determination to live started all the curative forces of his subconscious nature, and the ideal of life, "I will live," crowded out the expectation of death. He did live.

3. Some fresh light on the subject is also furnished by recent laboratory work which shows that mental suggestion in some form is the third great factor in this phenomena.

Our bodily tissue, as the scientists put it, is made up of cells, and in each cell is a nervous center, a minor seat of subconsciousness, which may be called the mind of the cell. The subconsciousness is the part of us to which we do not usually pay much attention, but which carries on all the natural functions when we are not thinking about them, or when we are asleep. Disease is the lethargy of the subconsciousness in any series or section of cell-minds, retarding the usual functions; and disease is cured by stimulating or vitalizing again these cell-minds. Now the special line of recent experiments is to ascertain the means of stimulating the cell-minds in the bodily tissue. It is found that what we call the curative power of drugs is merely the stimulating power and the directing power which certain drugs have on cell-mind. And also, it is found that in certain instances,—not in all, but in some instances, the same stimulus and direction that drugs give to the cell-mind can be given by stimulated mental force from the mind-center, through mental ideas or images.

This is fresh confirmation of an old truth, and helps to explain these cures that are effected by powdered biscuit, wooden magnets, Roman shrines, or Christian Science, in new stimulus through mental action.

We might mention even more marvelous instances of the power of mind over body as shown in cases of mind in hypnotic control;

but these we shall reserve for a later address when the power of mental suggestion and the appeal to the subconscious self are considered. But we may state briefly that this recent research emphasizes as never before that "the true physician is not a mere drug doctor; that his larger scope to-day involves, in the treatment of disease, not merely chemical forces in the body, but also psychic and ethical forces, which are operative in the body and as actual as any chemical agencies; that the study of the relation of mind and body is bringing new factors of health into view; that the new science of therapeutics will aim to treat where it is necessary, not a fraction of a man, but the integral man, and will incorporate into its diagnosis, in a larger and more scientific way than ever, the psychic and ethical factors in the case; and that in the newer medical curriculum, mind as well as body are to be more largely studied, and psychology is to have its place with physiology."

Hear this startling statement from Dr. Schofield: "The power of mind over the body has limits, but they have never yet been ascertained. All one can do to cure himself, the forces he can set in action, are as yet unknown, but they are far greater than most people imagine."

Nor is it the action of mere mind that we consider most important, although that must be trained and used along right lines. But it is the human mind when it is stimulated, strengthened, energized by the divine that is the most powerful agent in both moral and physical recovery. It is, as we shall later aim to show, mind reinforced by divine grace through faith and prayer that can accomplish the greatest results.

III. THE SPIRITUAL MASTERY OF THE BODY

THE spiritual mastery of the body, the force we call self-control, is not merely equipoise and mental equilibrium, but the dominance of the whole life by its highest power. It is not a discussion of theories, but a vital, practical fight, an earnest everyday striving for results. It is the mastery of the body for health and happiness.

How we love to see the dominance of mind in the world! How we love an invincible and dauntless spirit! How we admire even that pagan but courageous cry of the poet Henley:

> "I am the master of my fate,
> I am the captain of my soul!"

We recognize the right of mind over body. It is both fundamental and natural. It is both reasonable and divine. Perhaps we ought to say, most divinely reasonable. For it is the right of the spiritual over the natural; the right of the eternal over the transitory. This body in a few years will crumble into dust, but mind is immortal,—the spirit will live on forever.

We need not discuss the definitions of mind or spirit, nor revive the old contentions between dichotomy and trichotomy, that is, whether we are body and mind merely, or body, mind and spirit. It will suffice for our present discussion to recognize the great distinction between body and that incorporeal part of us, which is the seat of intelligence, emotions and will—call it what we may—mind, spirit, soul.

When God said to man in the beginning, "Have dominion!" he said it to man as the highest of all his creations. And when, in this highest creation, the command again goes forth, "Have dominion!" it is surely to the highest part in man,—his mind, his soul, his divine spirit.

We acknowledge the supremacy among human things of the human reason, the divine soul. We see constantly the great achievements of intelligence in the world. We see the marvelous products of mental efforts,—in works of invention, the accomplishments of great purposes and constructions, the achievements in literature, in science and art. We see the superb creations of human genius,—mind touched by the divine to its highest.

It has been taken generally for granted that while the wondrous powers of mind worked through the body and that the body must be kept in good condition for their working,—yet the body itself was largely independent of these powers and was not amenable to them in its own special workings. So that if the body was sick, it must be treated from without by external remedies, or by extraneous substances taken into the system.

The conclusion, however, in these days is irresistible, that the mind has great influence over the body, both in health and sickness, in more wonderful ways than we have sometimes dreamed. Some of this marvelous influence we have already noted.

Even more subtle than the mental influence on the bodily functions is the moral. This fact is coming into greater recognition as a scientific truth: the direct and intimate relations between sin and sickness, and between sickness and sin. Sometimes, in hereditary and other cases, it is sickness that is the cause of sin. But in most cases, and either personally or by heredity, it is sin that produces sickness. "Disorders of the body often flow from moral disorders; sickness may be sometimes the direct precipitation of sin; disease is sometimes merely the dregs of depravity." Every case, of course, demands separate and careful diagnosis. Often it is the sins of the father or the grandfather visited upon the children. Sometimes it is sin against the laws of health in former generations. But nearly always, in its last analysis, ill-health has a very close relation to sin.

There is truth in what Matthew Arnold says in his book, "Literature and Dogma": "Medical science has never gauged,—never, perhaps, enough set itself to gauge, the intimate connection between moral fault and disease. To what extent, or in how many cases, what is called illness is due to moral springs having been used amiss, whether by being over-used, or by not being used sufficiently, we hardly know at all and we too little inquire. Certainly, it is due to this very much more than we commonly think; and the more it is due to this, the more do moral therapeutics rise in possibility and importance. The bringer of light and happiness, the calmer and pacifier and stimulator, is one of the chiefest of doctors. Such a doctor was Jesus. Indications enough remain to show the line of the Master, His perceptions of the large part of moral cause in many kinds of disease and His method of addressing to this part His cure."

A thoughtful young physician said not long ago to a Christian minister: "I am sometimes disgusted with my work. I am expected to cure a man of disorders and diseases which may be largely the result of his evil appetites and passions, and then, without touching his soul, leave him to return again to wallow in his evil. All that I am doing, as I see it, is to undo the stern lessons whereby a man is taught, through suffering in the body, that he has sinned in the soul. I wish I could deliver him from the sin in his soul while I am delivering him from the suffering in his body."

Perhaps he puts the case too strongly; and yet, is there not a real truth in the feeling back of his words? Ought not even the ordinary physician be so familiar with the laws of mind and soul that he could suggest the secret causes and prescribe rational methods for their treatment? Many physicians are already doing this very thing with most helpful results. The inculcation, the inoculation of spiritual life, is a step higher than mental faith, and can be made most fruitful in therapeutic results.

And we ministers, if I may speak a word for my own profession, hail every real student in science, and especially every well-educated medical man, as our ally and fellow-worker in bringing in the kingdom of spiritual sanity and wholeness. As one thinker has well put it: "The healing of the body and the healing of the soul are different aspects of one and the same mystery of regeneration."

The chief value and strength of this new thought is the emphasis that it places upon cheerfulness, hopefulness and a perpetual and persistent optimism. It believes in God, it believes in Christ the active ideal in all things divinest; it believes in the Holy Spirit of encompassing love—and these are the great truths of life. It joyously emphasizes the health of God's countenance and what that belief may effect in the personal life. Many of us are persuaded that such a view will help to bring us all to a better frame of mind, to a healthier tone in religious life, to a more vigorous, a more militant faith in God and a less passive acquiescence in sickness and sin. And, therefore, for our everyday and ordinary life, whether we are sick or well, we call upon you to consider such specific things as these that follow, for such things as these make better conditions, both mental and physical. They tone up the system, help to give Nature a chance, cordially co-operate with all the medical care and treatment that may be given to you.

Thought-life is real life. "As a man thinketh in his heart, so is he." Thoughts are deeds. Thought is potential in both spirit and body.

What is referred to is the thinking that is the usual and habitual atmosphere of your mind. It means the thoughts which you constantly entertain, the thoughts in which you dwell, your habit of thought, your spirit of life, your views, your secret convictions and ambitions, your controlling ideals. These thoughts that take hold of a man's inmost life, and are the things that represent his own secret inner world—known only to himself and God. Such thoughts are *you*—your real vital self—the self that has the influence on your life and other lives.

This is the tremendous truth—being is

more important than doing. What you are is vastly more important than what you say or do. What you are is your thought, your affections—that whole inner, vital, palpitating life that is dominated by your mind.

Therefore, you have the duty and responsibility of right mental habits. Many of the ills of life are due to wrong thinking, to evil mental habits, and to the careless allowance of unwholesome mental moods. Sometimes you may imagine that you may think what you please if you do not allow the thoughts to escape into words or crystallize into deeds. But have you full liberty within the brain? Can you indulge yourself with impunity there? You do so at great peril. You can no more be careless of the inner life than of the outer. More careful must you be of the inner, for it is the source and fountain of the outer life. Therefore, be careful what sort of books you read, be careful as to your companions and associations. Beware of anything that breeds doubt, evil thoughts, ignoble desires and false ambitions. Cultivate everything that breeds nobleness in the soul. The Master holds us responsible in the spirit of our lives. These thoughts of ours are innocent or guilty before God. Your thought counts, and counts vastly. Your thought is you.

This is not merely important in a spiritual way—it is also vastly important in a physical way that we should be pure-minded and healthy-minded in our thinking.

We are fully responsible for the thoughts we entertain. We are not responsible for the random thoughts that come flitting in and out, but the thoughts that we hold and dwell on. We are not always responsible for random thoughts, but we are for the thoughts we cherish. As a quaint old writer once said: "We cannot help the birds flying over our heads, but we can prevent them building nests in our hair."

Paul recognized that we could control our thought. This is what that sacred teaching to the Philippians meant when it said: "Whatsoever things are true, whatsoever things are honest, whatsoever things are just, whatsoever things are pure, whatsoever things are of good report: if there be any virtue, if there be any praise, think on these things."

Further, you have the duty of asserting your potentialities. You are made for health and happiness. Never forget it. You were created as a child of God. Live up to your birthright. You are in God's thought and love a nobler being than you are living at present—you have a greater power than you are exercising, you can render a fuller service to yourself and humanity and God than you have as yet dreamed. The thoughts of your heart make the deeds of your life. Our thoughts do not end with the thinking. Thought is power, and has its issue in reality. Every thought leaves its impress within as without. Every thought leaves its indelible record within. "I am a part of all that I have met," Tennyson wrote in his Ulysses. And all that we have thought also becomes a part of us. Every evil thought degrades us and stains and scars the fiber of our soul. But every good thought is a new strength and blessing to the soul. A noble soul is built up of noble thoughts.

There is no limit to the effect of good thinking, when it is backed by your will and crowned by the grace of God. Can it restore to health? It can, in many instances, and it can do greater things.

You have the duty and responsibility of realizing that your spirit is made for conquest, because it is in loving fellowship with the divine spirit. We do not half realize our powers. When we are leagued with God, all things are possible. We can be more than conquerors, when we are leagued with God. By a covenant of consecration and faith, we are taking hold of the sources of omnipotence.

Most marvelous work has been accomplished in this world by those who in the power of God have lived their lives and have done their deeds. The supreme mind in this world is the mind of Christ. And yet—listen to this appeal: "Let this mind be in you which was also in Christ Jesus." These are audacious words, but they express a great truth and a living possibility. Something of that mind which was in Christ Jesus, you may have, if you ask God for it—so that you may think some of His great thoughts after Him. The mind of Jesus was purity, humility, nobility, divinity. The mind of Jesus was wise with a heavenly wisdom and warm with a divine love.

Let a man think in the spirit of Jesus, let a man speak in the spirit of Jesus, let a man live in the spirit of Jesus and that man is a victor over the body.

A man who has the ideal of Jesus dwelling

in his thoughts continually, will have there the inspiration of the noblest living. His thoughts cannot dwell in that atmosphere of goodness, without, by very contagion, becoming infected with divine ambition. His love can transform the heart; His ideals can inspire the mind and life until we, beholding as in a glass the glory of the Lord, shall be gradually transformed into the same image, even from glory to glory.

Such a mind, divine and dominant in us, will accomplish God's purpose in us and by us. It will undoubtedly help us in our fight for physical health and it will be conquering power in our fight for spiritual health. This gives the invincible spirit, this gives the note of absolute conquest in all things—the sense of eternal union with the love of God from which nothing can separate us.

SECOND CONFERENCE

The Therapeutic Value of Faith and Prayer

I. Faith as a Vital Force.
II. The Healing Value of Prayer.

I. FAITH AS A VITAL FORCE

FAITH and prayer are often considered merely as spiritual factors. We want to show in this address that they have also physical and therapeutic value.

There is a great deal in that phrase that Tolstoi uses in one of his books—"Faith is the force of life." For, in fact, faith is more than spiritual imagination or spiritual comprehension. It is a vital energy. It is not merely the power that relates the finite to the infinite, that bridges the gulf between the seen and the unseen, but it is a stimulus to all the latent faculties of life. It is as large and as real a factor in our lives as reason, or will, or the affections. It is a basal principle of life, and we ought to recognize it as such.

Every modern physician uses more or less of faith in his practice. It is a necessary part of his work—as important as his drugs. He must inspire faith and confidence, in his patients; otherwise his service is not effective. If a patient have faith in his doctor, the medicine does more good; in truth, if patient have strong faith in the doctor, the cure is sometimes effected without medicine. Some medicines and treatment, as given by great physicians in whom people have faith, may have no effect when administered in the identical way by another physician who has no faith in himself and in whom his patient has no faith.

All the various modern cults of healing—faith cure, mental healing, so-called Christian Science, and the more recent Emmanuel Movement, emphasize faith, and rightly so, as a prime necessity in their work. Some, however, depend on faith entirely and in most illogical and undiscriminating ways; others, such as the Emmanuel Movement, in a more sensible and rational way.

We may recall the historical fact that the early church continued for some time the apostolic work of healing, and its practice consisted largely of faith and prayer. It is an interesting chapter in the history of the church as recorded in fragmentary pages of early Christian literature.

It is refreshing to find the modern church coming back again to a realization that it has a certain part, at least, in helping both the souls and bodies of men, and in understanding that its mission is not to disembodied spirits, but to the whole life in the body.

We recognize that in material affairs, as in spiritual, the man with faith is the man who brings about results. "Faith," as one says, "is behind the great achievements of our modern life. Faith is the keystone of success. Without faith we do the work of life with lagging hearts. With it our powers are at their best. Chronic doubt kills effort and cripples its powers. But faith—not credulity, not rashness—but honest, constructive faith which realizes by action that 'assurance of things hoped for,'—such a force will carry us over mountains of difficulty and leave us fresh for the next climb."

Faith is thus a daily principle in business and in social life. We must have faith in our fellows to some large extent, or business stops, and social life becomes a mockery. Faith is also a principle which is used in science. We think of science as based on knowledge. So it is. It goes usually only as far as the five senses take it, and yet it believes further than it sees. It has never actually seen the essence of life, only its manifestations in electricity or the other energies. But it has faith in these, so that the whole universe becomes intelligent and understandable.

Faith is, of course, a chief principle in religion and it gives the basis of action there. Doubt paralyzes, but faith gives the vital touch of reality and is the means of progress toward all higher things.

Now extend this same principle into the therapeutic field. As a matter of fact, it is being more and more recognized that in all mental and spiritual methods of dealing with disease, faith is a powerful factor. "After all," as Dr. Osler says, "faith is a great leveler of life. Without it, man can do nothing; with it, even with a fragment, as a grain of mustard seed, all things are possible to him. Faith in us, faith in our drugs and methods, is the great stock in trade of the profession. . . . It is the aurum potabile, the touchstone of success in medicine. As Galen says, 'Confidence and hope do more good than physic.' He cures most in whom most are confident."

But in this special work it may be asked: What kind of faith is needed for the therapeutic work? And we may answer that it is not a superstitious faith that is needed, nothing blind, arbitrary or unreasoning; nor a theological faith or creed. Indeed, people of widely different creeds, and of no creed, are equally helped in this movement. Nor is it a stultifying faith, believing without evidence and affirming belief of what, in your inmost soul, you are not persuaded. Instead it is a simple, reasonable, fundamental faith—an attitude of life and soul which means reverence, willingness, obedience. That is enough to begin with, and it will increase. It means such a faith as this:

1. Faith in God's love and His loving purpose towards us. For God is love, life, health. He wills health for us. He helps us to health, as far as we allow Him. He is opposed to pain and disease and abnormality, as He is opposed to vice and sin.

2. Faith in the healing power of Nature (which is another name for God). Nature is always seeking to heal us. Take away the barriers; give Nature a chance and she will heal.

3. Faith in ourselves when our wills and energies are stimulated, strengthened, and energized by God's grace. We must stir up the gift that is in us. The power is often

latent. It needs the stimulus of new exertion; it needs re-education.

Such a faith is deeper and larger than belief. Belief is accepting a thing by our reason. Faith is accepting by our whole life—involving consecration and obedience. Belief only needs the mind; faith needs mind, affections, will,—the whole being.

As a matter of fact, we do not need many definite beliefs for therapeutic help; but we do need this firm and abiding faith in God and His love, and His gracious purposes, and our own power of response to Him.

A recent writer has said: "A great deal of alleged physical suffering is primarily mental. A great many people have 'fixed ideas' of disease, pain, debility, fatigue, dread, inefficiency, and inexpressible woes. Much oftener than we realize, these can be transplanted without surgery or medication. I do not mean that they are not real suffering. They are as real as the grave. But they are not grounded in physical infirmity, and they are not to be cured by physic. The mind becomes possessed of a conviction that a certain part of the body is infirm, and imputes pain to that part in spite of all the medicine in the world. Hundreds of people refuse to get well after the physician has cured them. It is not his fault, and it is not their fault; they have simply had disease suggested to them until they cannot think at all except upon that assumption." *

And for such conditions, the stimulus of a new faith, and the re-education of the whole mental outlook are needed. As Dr. Lewellys F. Barker says: "The patient afflicted with a so-called 'functional' nervous disorder must, it is true, believe in his physician, but the physician's task is to re-educate the patient to believe in himself. More than half the ills of one class of nervous patients depend upon a loss of confidence in their own ability, upon a sense of past failure and of future impotency. They have tried to do things outside their powers, and, having failed, have become convinced that they cannot in any way be efficient. Their minds are concentrated upon their failures and their disabilities instead of upon their successes. It is necessary to teach them how again to become confident and self-reliant; by assigning to them small tasks, well within their powers, and proving to them that they are capable of overcoming difficulty after difficulty. Many

* Max Eastman in *Atlantic Monthly*, May, 1900.

may soon be taught to count victories where formerly every effort spelled defeat."*

This is the interesting point. Modern science, as expressed in the fullest studies in physiology and psychology, also emphasizes this same need of faith. Physiology shows the wonderful power of faith in its action on the bodily functions and organs. Fear, for example, can distort and retard nerves and functions and upset the whole life. Faith can steady and stimulate and harmonize the whole life—the nerves and all the bodily functions. Psychology similarly in all its studies shows how faith can stimulate and transform mental moods and awaken latent energies.

We see, therefore, that the principle that the Master used in His work, both in healing the body and in healing the soul—the fundamental principle of faith as a prime necessity of healing, is the very one that it has been found necessary to use all through the centuries, whenever healing work has been done. The same thing holds true to-day.

We see also the reason for it. The Master was using no arbitrary methods, but spiritual laws, divinely written by God in our very

* Introd. to Prof. Oppenheim's *Letters on Psychotherapeutics.*

being. In order to accomplish similar results, we also must use these same laws, so far as we can, and come back to the very first principles of the method of the Master. We are getting to fundamental ground as we follow Him, who was and is the Great Physician of the Body and Soul.

"Faith," as Bishop Fallows says, "is a dynamic power within the soul itself. It springs from the innermost nature. It can be reinforced and strengthened from without, but must ever originate from within. In the healing of the mind or body, the energy exerted by the patient himself upon himself is of the utmost importance. It must begin with the belief that he can be helped. He may say, 'I have no faith,' when he seeks relief, but the very fact that he seeks it is the clear indication that he has some faith. According to the measure of his faith will be the corresponding good."

Faith is essential. The patient cannot merely sit down and wait and be healed. In mental medicine, he has something to do, and a great deal. He must exert himself; he must have faith and obey. If a man would have help along these lines, he must give up the doubting mood, and come in the eager and expectant mood, hoping for good. He must give up the critical mood, captious of everything that is said or done, and come in the hospitable mood, keeping mind and heart open. He must give up the selfish mood, thinking only of self and his troubles, and let his thoughts go out to others, sympathizing with them, and hoping and praying for them. He must stop thinking merely of the body, and come into thoughts of the soul, of the divine life, of God and His loving purposes.

Christianity in the largest sense is health, spiritual, mental, physical. Holiness and wholesomeness are from the same roots in etymology and in divine sources. The words that John writes in his third epistle are suggestive: "Brethren, I desire above all things that thou shalt prosper, and be in health, even as thy soul prospereth."

Men must be taught to exorcise and cast out the demons of fear, fret, weakness and worry. Such things are altogether evil and antagonistic to the best Christian life. People must be taught not to give up to sickness but to resist it, just as they resist sin, and they must avoid temptations to sickness, as they would avoid temptations to sin.

The church is beginning to protest against

ailments forming the bulk of conversation when the subject of the weather gives out. The church ought to protest against the luxury of grief in which some indulge with loss of interest in life and neglect of duties.

The church ought to protest against worry and fret. John Wesley wrote in one of his journals: "I would as soon curse and swear as worry. It is doubting God." We ought to have more of pure, strong, simple, brave Christianity, with apostolic joyousness and apostolic power! We ought to have the joyous early Christian mood of the disciples with our faces perpetually to the sunshine!

What we need in our churches is a more virile belief and practice. There is a place for the passive virtues and for quiescent faith and for gentle acquiescence, but it must not predominate nor monopolize. Religion is in danger of being emasculated by resignation. We need more of the spirit of resistance,—resistance unto blood. We need a manlier type of thought. We need a sturdier emphasis on the stronger, more vigorous, and healthier elements. The gospel is not weakness, but power; not sickness, but health; not weeping, but laughter and shoutings. We need to feel with Sidney

Lanier: "My Lord is large; my Lord is strong."

What is called "religious experience" has very close relations with the whole life,—spiritual, mental and physical. It is the progressive awakening to the consciousness of God with us, of His wondrous power encompassing us and uplifting us. There is a profound philosophy in it. It is the process by which a man gets a new point of view, new ideals, a new allegiance for the life. It takes us away from self, from doubts, from symptoms. It puts before us an image of purity and power, of holiness and health. It calls us with all the love of our heart and all the strength of our soul to be like the Master in His life and spirit. It gives us a living ideal—God's own perfect ideal for us. The ideals that we create in our own minds may be weak, wrong, imperfect, inadequate. But here is the finest and noblest that human heart can conceive, and that divine love can offer.

Here we are at the fountain head. We are at the source of life and strength. God created; God can renew. We can become increasingly one with Him and it will mean infinitely to us, both in holiness and health.

A serene spirit, a quiet heart, and a confident faith in God, are substantial helps to the preservation or restoration of that mental equipoise which must always come before physical equilibrium is assured.

II. THE HEALING VALUE OF PRAYER

THESE thoughts on faith, as a vital force, lead naturally to a consideration of an allied subject,—the therapeutic value of prayer. In his "Varieties of Religious Experience," Professor James says: "As regards prayer for the sick, if any medical fact can be considered to stand firm, it is that in certain environments, prayer may contribute to recovery, and should be encouraged as a therapeutic measure."

There are many to whom prayer in these days is a perplexity, rather than a joy and a strength. It is so often kept down on a low level as a mere business transaction between God and us, that all its deeper philosophy is left to seem unreasonable and its divinest meaning is made obscure. Yet prayer is the supreme experience in human life. We are indebted to science for clearing away much that is unreasonable in the modern thought of prayer, and also for reassuring us of the scientific facts and analogies of the seeming miracles that can be wrought by intelligence in ordinary life, and which point, as we shall show later, to a Supreme Intelligence that works in His universe, and gives us by a thousand manifestations the assurance that "more things are wrought by prayer, than this world dreams of."

The greatest power of prayer, however, is not in its possible answers in the material realm, nor in awful times of special emergency. Its greatest power is in bringing us continually into soothing and strengthening contact with the divine, that our wills may be brought into harmony with God, and that there may come into our souls new strength for accomplishing God's work by our own heart and hands. Prayer is communion, privilege, companionship.

There are many speculative difficulties in the subject of prayer, if we chose to consider them, and especially when we view prayer on its material side. It would seem as if the acceptance of natural law were full of questionings and invincible arguments against the material response to prayer. But the philosophy of prayer cannot be discussed by mere logic-chopping. Prayer is the supremest experience in the human life; it is "the stoop of the soul that upraises it, too"; and its deepest philosophy has never been fathomed, nor ever can be, by the scientific method or the logic of pure reason.

We cannot restrict the possible power of prayer, even in the way of material response. It may help us on this point to remember that this universe is not a machine, set in motion under fixed laws and left to itself. There is a supreme living personality in this world,—God in His world, working out His purposes toward "one far-off divine event to which the whole creation moves,"—and what we call natural laws, are merely His customary modes of action. He is not a prisoner in the chains of His own laws; He is supreme even in natural laws. And a supreme intelligence, if it will, can so use these laws as to bring about results that of themselves would not occur. And He does.

You have noticed sometimes what effect mere human intelligence has in so using natural laws to bring about new results. Electricity, for instance, is a natural agent under natural laws, and in itself is useless, or means lightning and destruction. But man modifies these natural forces, he adapts them to a purpose, and the electricity serves him and does his bidding over land and under seas. It runs to the farthest parts of earth with his messages. "In forty minutes, it circles the globe." It lights his streets, it drives his engines, it even cures his diseases. Man has not changed a single natural law, but by adapting these forces under these laws, he has made them serve a new purpose. Cannot God do this, as man has done, and even on a larger scale?

Ordinary sunlight, to give another illustration, has its natural laws, and man cannot change them. But he can so modify and use them, that what sunlight would not do without the cunning mind of man, now it will do, and will paint for him lifelike pictures in black and white, and even in colors. Has a miracle been wrought by the process of photography? No natural law has been changed, but intelligence has so controlled natural law that a new purpose has been wrought and a new thing accomplished.

Perchance you may wake in the morning with a sore throat. You have been careless or negligent, and have caught cold, and natural law is at work. If nothing is done, natural law may take its course, and the cold may develop into something worse. But immediately you set about to modify the natural process of law by bringing into operation other natural laws. You apply counter-irritants or other remedies, and before the day is over intelligent action has conquered and the disease has been averted. Natural law has been used in new ways by other natural laws through human intelligence and action. Cannot Divine Intelligence do the same and greater? And in these ways, God does work.

If we did not understand these everyday things that we mention, we might call them miraculous, but since we understand them, we say it is intelligence at work. May it not be that results which we may call miraculous are wrought for us by God merely through the infinite and all-wise action of a Supreme Intelligence,—and results that, without prayer, might not have come to pass?

In all these things, let us remember that no prayer is answered unless the man who prays works with God toward its answer. That petition that we pray every day, "Give us this day our daily bread," amounts to nothing if the man prays it and sits down to eat with folded arms. If the prayer means anything, it means that the man is willing to work with God to effect the answer.

Prayer must not in the least be allowed to take the place of human effort and responsibility. If a great battle is at stake, we must pray earnestly to the God of Battles, but keep our powder dry. If our house is on fire, we must not kneel down and pray, but pray as we run with the water-buckets. If we want a good harvest, we must pray, but be sure of our grain and the right sowing-time. If we want business success, we must pray, but also work with all our might. God has not given us the privilege of prayer in order to cut the nerve of effort or to put a premium on indolence. Therefore, in the same way, if we pray for health, we must use every sensible and legitimate method to secure it, and we must be willing to fulfill the conditions and laws of health, so far as we know, or our prayer is not a true prayer.

Another thing must be considered. No prayer is answered by what we call miracle, where natural means and natural laws are sufficient for the answer. God respects the eternal laws that He has made—His own best ways—and He will not controvert them. It is futile to expect it. But times may occur in the divine economy of the ages, when prayer is answered by what seems to us a miracle, although it is but the natural law of God. But the notion in some minds that God is all the time playing fast and loose with His own laws in order to gratify the prayers of His children seems presumptuous and preposterous.

Would we have it, forsooth, that, for our own wish or convenience or the working out of our plans, God should reverse His laws? True it is, as we said, that God knows His own laws—that He can modify at His wisdom everything but the essential ethical laws of His own being. But is it not the more reasonable to suppose that in most cases prayer merely brings about new results through these same laws of God, and leads us unto fuller harmony with God, fuller obedience to His laws, and hence conquest in them. No natural law is controverted under ordinary circumstances in answer to prayer. But natural law is used by divine intelligence, or we are so inspired, as to effect new results.

In a word, then, while we may hold that no prayer changes any law of God, or natural law, nor alters God's will—we also hold that every honest prayer is answered, and that every honest prayer has in it not only longing and desire, but a willingness to work with God toward the answer of the prayer.

Thus far, however, we have been considering what we may call the ordinary or the lower aspects of prayer. They are important, and we have dwelt on them in some measure in order to bring into contrast the higher meaning of prayer. This greatest power of prayer is the power that it has of bringing us continually into such soothing and strengthening contact with the divine that our wills are brought into harmony with God, and there comes into our souls new strength for accomplishing God's work by our own hearts and hands. In this fact is also found the special and greatest therapeutic value of prayer, as we come into this higher meaning—beyond petition into communion.

As an eminent writer has put it: "Prayer has a regenerating and uplifting effect on character; but in affecting character it must also affect the nervous system. It does not seem irrational to believe that prayer opens the inner consciousness to the absorption of spiritual energy. This attitude of receptivity toward the higher things in turn affects life and character and the calmed and purified spirit acts on the nervous organization, restoring its tone and rhythm."

Now in all our thought of prayer, remember that we stand to God, not externally, not as distantly calling some far-off Being. "It is not," as one says, "like calling up a person by a long-distance 'phone and then waiting for material gifts." But we must remember that in God we live and move and have our being—"we are organically related to God, we exist in Him spiritually as thoughts exist in our minds." And when we pray sincerely and earnestly, our prayer arises to God as a thought arises in our minds. Such a thought sometimes takes possession of us. So real prayer may take possession of us. A real prayer may also take possession of God and bring blessing.

Tennyson saw this higher meaning of prayer when he said: "Prayer is like opening a sluice between the great ocean and our little channels when the great sea gathers itself together and flows in at full tide."

It is often the case that those nervously afflicted cannot put their prayer into words. They cannot command their thoughts or words as they wish. For these, it is most helpful oftentimes, if they follow a form of prayer,—simple, definite, uplifting.

But it is not always necessary that prayer should be in words. Just the attitude of communion and trust is often the most helpful and uplifting. It is the prayer of silence and trust. It is just going into a quiet spot and waiting on God. It is the way of the Mystics, the Quietists, the Friends. But it is a good way. As the Scriptures say: "Be still and know that I am God."

"One of the most beautiful forms of autosuggestion," as Bishop Fallows points out, "is prayer. Not that auto-suggestion is the whole of prayer. It is rather our preparation for the effects of prayer. Through its use we push away for a time from ourselves the engrossing preoccupation that shuts out higher interests, we open, as it were, a hidden door in our consciousness through which come new life and power and energy from God."

Such a practice as this—silent waiting befor God for half an hour a day in the quiet—relaxed, passive, but with the windows of the soul open, will be oftentimes most helpful to the nervous sufferer. It helps to produce that quiet and serenity of spirit that is most desired. It opens in some mystic but real way, an actual connection between the soul and uplifting spiritual forces. Prayer, in this way, passively and without words, but full of thanksgiving and trust in God, brings new strength and help.

Prayer before sleep has distinct therapeutic value. The mechanism of sleep is unknown, but it is more than the cessation of consciousness. Many beneficial physical changes take place during sleep. Waste is repaired; functions reorganized. Often a ten minute nap is a tonic and a medicine, better than food or drink; renewing the mental and physical life. Sleep is largely a matter of suggestion, inhibition and control. Very important upon sleep and dreams and the deepest life are the last thoughts before going to sleep at night. Here is the value of prayer, when used just before sleeping. It is a scientific, physical help as well as spiritual.

"The fundamental religious point," as a noted psychologist says, "is that in prayer spiritual energy, which would otherwise slumber, does become active, and spiritual work of some kind is really effected. This means, not only that prayer makes us better men and women, but that the spiritual energy which it brings may be translated into acts which give us more force as working beings, more power of achievement, more influence in the social order."

The therapeutic value of prayer may thus be considered as resting fundamentally in these facts:

1. Prayer brings the mind into a quiet and trustful attitude, and this reacts on the body.

2. Prayer is the continually hopeful spirit and this helps physical condition.

3. Prayer stimulates us to help ourselves to co-operate in the answer to prayer.

4. Prayer is sometimes directly answered in physical healing.

5. Prayer unites the human forces to the divine forces.

6. Prayer is the opening of the sluices of the soul for the divine inflowing.

7. Prayer is the atmosphere in which the divine Spirit of life lives and works.

In view of all this, it were folly to tell people that it is their duty to pray. Duty is too cold a word. Privilege and glory are the only words to connect with prayer. It is possible, however, that, through the first impulse of duty, a way may be made into the sanctuary of privilege.

Those who know what prayer means find in it joyous companionship in solitude; it means genial sympathy in the recoil from the coldness of life; it means the delicious satisfaction of thought and feeling in the loving closeness of a living presence. More than that, prayer means the uplifting of the heart and mind into a higher atmosphere, into the living communion with the divine life and love.

A remarkable declaration and confirmation of this position concerning the value of prayer as a means to mental health, is that of Dr. Murray Hyslop, physician superintendent of the Royal Hospitals, Bridewell and Bethlehem, in London: "As an alienist and one whose whole life has been concerned with the sufferings of the human mind," he says, "I would state that of all the hygienic measures to counteract disturbed sleep, depression of spirits, and all the miserable sequels of a distressed mind, I would undoubtedly give the first place to the simple habit of prayer. Let there be but a habit of nightly communion, not as a mendicant, nor repeater of words, but as an humble individual who submerges or asserts his individuality as an integral part of a greater whole. Such a habit does more to cleanse the spirit and strengthen the soul to overcome mere incidental emotionalism than any other therapeutic agent known to me."

One who has found the secret of prayer, one who has learned its solace, its richness of joy, its hidden fountains of strength—believes in prayer, rejoices in prayer, although he cannot see that a single one of his prayers ever receives an answer in a tangible form. He has risen far above that aspect of prayer. He does not limit or measure the divine by his own human desires or expectations. He believes and knows that every one of his prayers is answered, because he believes in God and knows an infinitely loving, wise Good Heart, even the Heart of God. That Heart, he is sure, hears him and loves him and will do whatsoever is best for him.

One has aptly put it: "Perhaps we are like wireless stations, each tuned to the vibrations that individualize us, with God the Almighty Center holding the key for every human being. . . . Our connection with God, the source of all life, is never broken, it is true; but prayer is the live current which makes that connection efficient. Without prayer, we are isolated, as it were, at the end of a dead wire. The universe itself is, to the devout mind, founded upon prayer, that is, on the principle of dependence, which is the fundamental note of prayer. Science and psychology concur in such a view. The world we live in, great as it seems to us, is as a grain of sand to the bulk of a vast mountain when compared to the numberless orbs that revolve through the million miles of space. But law and order govern the whole. Part is dependent upon part. We seem to ourselves, perhaps, isolated and self-contained. Yet I lift my hand, I make the slightest motion, and the clearest-headed thinker in the world of science tells me that the very movement of my fingers sends its vibrations to the farthest star, for hundreds of millions, or billions or quadrillions or sextillions of miles. Distance makes no difference. There can be no motion in one part without motion being in some way felt in another." *

Such is the power of prayer,—a real thing in life, a real force in this universe.

* Bishop Samuel Fallows, in *Health and Happiness*, 1908.

THIRD CONFERENCE

Possibilities in the Control of Subconsciousness

I. Glimpses of the Subconscious Self.
II. The Training of the Hidden Energies.

I. GLIMPSES OF THE SUBCONSCIOUS SELF

DR. OLIVER WENDELL HOLMES makes the observation: "We all have a double, who is wiser and better than we are, and who puts thoughts into our heads, and words into our mouths. Do we not all commune with our own hearts upon our beds? Do we not all divide ourselves, and go as buffets on questions of right or wrong, of wisdom or folly? Who or what is it that resolves the stately parliament of the day, with all its forms and conventionalities and pretences, and the great Me presiding, into the committee of the whole, with Conscience in the chair, that holds its solemn session through the watches of the night?"*

Of course, the first question in our consideration of this subject is, What is the subconscious self? We may answer by asking some other question. What is it that carries on all

* *Mechanism in Thought and Morals,* 1869.

the functions of life while we are unconscious of their action? We go to sleep, and our inner life goes on perfectly, the beating of the heart, the circulation of the blood, the digestion, the breathing of the lungs. We are put to sleep by chloroform or ether, or by hypnotism. The inner life still continues its subtle workings. Perhaps some slight modifications may be noted, due to the anæsthetic, but the great functions go on uninterruptedly. We are injured in some way. We may be unconscious, yet the inner powers begin immediately to retrieve the injury. An innumerable army of tiny healers begin their work in our bodies. Who sets them to work?

What is the inner power that is used, for instance, when habit becomes second nature? When we learn our music so that we can talk or think independently as we play; or learn to carry on at the same time two separate lines of thought? What gives the power to some untaught mathematical genius, or to the musical prodigy known as Blind Tom?

What is the inner power that takes note of time and things, even when we are unconscious? We want to wake at a certain time —we have it on our minds, and we wake at the very hour. It is not the working of our conscious mind, for that is asleep. Is there a mind that never sleeps?

Various fire-alarms sound in the fire station. But the firemen so accustom themselves that they hear only their own special alarm. What is it that listens for this special alarm, and discriminates between this and the others?

What is the inner power of inspiration that brings forth great poems, music and other works of creation? These things seem to flow from our inner being.

What is the strange gift of unconscious cerebration? We have a problem; we leave it for awhile. Then, meantime, it somehow clears up. Or we have a subject to think over; we give it a week in our mind, with no particular conscious thought. Then we take it up and find that a great mass of related subjects have accumulated around it.

Where is the depository of memory? For, as a matter of fact, we remember everything that we have learned. We remember it, but we cannot always recall it. But special times or emergencies show it that it is all there, somewhere, in unconsciousness.

This classic instance is told by Coleridge: A German servant girl about twenty-five years old was taken ill with fever, and in her delirium, she cited long passages in Latin, Greek and Hebrew. Scholars were called in to hear this miracle. But later the marvel was explained. Years before she had lived in a minister's family. He was accustomed to recite his classics out loud. She had heard them; unconsciously it was all recorded. Memory never forgets an impression.

Confessions of those who have been almost drowned confirm the same phenomena. The whole life comes up before them in an instant—all its long-forgotten details. Memory's tablets are ineffaceable. Nevertheless two-thirds, if not seven-eighths, of these records are in the unconscious regions of mind.

These instances at least prove the existence of the region of the unconscious, and they suggest its remarkable possibilities, such as the dual self, and the triple or multiple personality and its problems.

The usual nomenclature of the conscious and the unconscious self is merely a convenient one, not strictly scientific. Psychology and even medical science are not all agreed as to terms. Some hold to the phrase " dissociation of consciousness" as more accurate. The general position of psychology holds to the unity of mind, although we may designate the two regions of the mind by different names. Prof. William James of Harvard, one of our leading psychologists, contends for the phrase "the unconscious mind" and what it represents. The name however is varied by different writers and is almost interchangeably called unconscious mind, subconscious mind, subjective mind, or subliminal self. Even these terms may each be differentiated. We shall use in this address that generally accepted term "the subconscious self," which Dr. Waldstein uses in his famous treatise on the subject.

It is interesting to recall that brilliant address of Dr. Oliver Wendell Holmes, on "Mechanism in Thought and Morals," delivered at Harvard just forty years ago, in which he asks the question: "Do we ever think without knowing that we are thinking? The question may be disguised so as to look a little less paradoxical. Are there any mental processes of which we are unconscious at the time, but which we recognize as having taken place by finding certain results in our minds? That there are such unconscious mental actions is laid down in the strongest terms by Leibnitz, whose doctrine reverses the axiom of Descartes into 'sum, ergo cogito.' The existence of unconscious thought is maintained by him in terms we might fairly call audacious, and illustrated by some of the most striking facts bearing upon it. The 'insensible perceptions,' he says, are as important in pneumatology as corpuscles are in physics. 'It does not follow,' he says again, 'that, because we do not perceive thought, it does not exist.' Something goes on in the mind which answers to the circulation of the blood and all the internal movements of the viscera. In one word, it is a great source of error to believe that there are no perceptions in the mind but those of which it is conscious."

He adds: "This is surely a sufficiently explicit and peremptory statement of the doctrine, which, under the names of 'latent consciousness,' 'obscure perceptions,' 'the hidden soul,' 'unconscious cerebration,' 'reflex action of the brain,' has been of late years emerging into general recognition in treatises of psychology." Now these words of Dr. Holmes' were written forty years ago. There is nothing new under the sun.

Some have assumed as a working hypothsis "that man possesses two minds, the subjective mind being, according to this view, the soul. But mind is one. All the phenomena connected with various so-called personalities in the same individual have been ultimately resolved into the one indivisible, normal self." Wundt, the founder of experimental psychology and the leader of the "new psychology," has announced his conviction of "the indivisible unity and inner oneness of the mental life in all its phases."

The unity of the mind, Dr. Alfred T. Schofield, of London, maintains, is a truth as needful to lay hold of as the unity of the body. Professor William James agrees with him when he says: "As the action of the mental factor in disease is unconscious, it cannot be recognized as mental by those who limit mind to consciousness. The word mind must, therefore, be extended to include all psychic action. Almost all the action of the mind upon the body as a factor in disease or in therapeutics is exercised subconsciously, automatically, and—perhaps often of necessity—unconsciously."

Now the fact of the subconscious self reminds us that there is a region of the unknown in mind and in religion, and in all life. We cannot escape from mystery in mind or religion or in medicine. A religion without its profound secrets is no religion; for it is not true. A science that has discovered all will never be known. Nor is mind to be excepted from the region of the unconscious or unfathomable.

Nevertheless there have already been certain things learned about this subconscious self that are most interesting and important. Some of these facts have been discovered concerning the subconscious mind by the careful and scientific investigators of the region of the subconscious by means of hypnotic condition. Such condition is often used to advantage in medical work.

A few words concerning this method may not be amiss in explaining its relation to the general subject of rational psychotherapy, which is our chief consideration.

Physicians in these days are studying and working along these lines with fruitful results. One of the clearest statements of this is in Dr. Albert Moll's work on "Hypnotism" in the chapter on Medical Aspects of Hypnotism. He says, to quote two or three brief paragraphs: "I think that hardly any of the newest discoveries are so important to the art of healing, apart from surgery, as the study of mental or hypnotic suggestion. . . . Suggestion will not again disappear from the foreground in medicine. . . . Suggestion will not supplant other methods of healing, but complete them. Now that it has been proved that organic changes can be caused by suggestion, we are obliged to ascribe a much greater importance to mental influences than we have hitherto done; . . . Suggestion is not only the key to the origin and aggravation of certain maladies, it also in some measure explains the working of drugs. . . . If medicines have different effects, when prescribed by different doctors, we shall not find the cause of this in chemical differences; we should rather ask if the manner of the prescription, the impression made by the doctor, and other mental factors, have not had some effect?"

The theory that hypnotism is due to a magnetic fluid is exploded. The theory that hypnotism is only possible in case of weak or diseased nerves is also discarded. We have learned that hypnotism is possible in healthy and normal subjects; that the hypnotic sleep differs only in cause and degree from the normal sleep, and that its greatest value is the influence on subconsciousness or subjective mind by the process of mental suggestion, a process which has more or less of permanent effect.

So that we can understand something further of what Dr. Moll means in his work on Hypnotism, when he says: "We have already seen what Bernheim and Liebault think, that hypnotism means suggestion, and suggestion is truly the chief agent in it. Bernheim's definition of hypnotism makes its therapeutic value more comprehensible. He believes that hypnosis is a particular mental state, in which susceptibility to suggestion is heightened. It follows from this that susceptibility exists apart from hypnosis; one is the natural complement of the other. . . . The therapeutics of suggestion," he continues, "are founded on the premise that a number of diseases can be cured or relieved merely by making the patient believe he will soon be better, and by firmly implanting this conviction in his mind. . . . If suggestion is to succeed, the patient must firmly believe that he is to be cured. . . . I should think it right, in certain cases, to send patients to some miracle-working spot. That Charcot was convinced of the healing power of faith is well known. It cannot be denied that faith and emotional excitement produce many results at Lourdes."

It is interesting to find in the recent treatise by Dr. Louis Waldstein, of New York, on "The Subconscious Self," many careful conclusions which are particularly pertinent in this connection. For instance, he says: "All the phenomena of so-called hypnotism can be referred to suggestion. The hypnotic condition, as well as what happens during its continuance, is suggested. With this step, the inquiry ceases to be confined to abnormal and ultra-critical regions, and thereby enters the domain of the ordinary processes of mental activity, and so brings the subject within a more easily obtainable reach. The hypnotic condition, hence, is a phase of the mind differing only in degree from the normal. . . ." And again, and this is most important: *"In many cases, it is not necessary to induce hypnotic sleep in order to influence subconscious conditions.* For instance, I am sure that suggestions methodically made before ordinary sleep would act quite as well as if made during hypnosis, and much good would result from a careful elaboration of such a method of treatment."

So also Dr. Halleck in his treatise on "The Education of the Central Nervous System," writes: "The highest medical authorities agree that mental attention strongly directed to any part of the body will produce physical change. If the attention is centered on the stomach, the digestion will suffer; if on the liver, that will become deranged. The vascularity of bodily organs and the caliber of the blood vessels can thus be made to undergo a change. In short, the physical results of mental attention are strongly marked."

To summarize briefly: The modern investigations of physiological psychology, what may be called the laboratory work of the science, are showing us in hitherto unsuspected ways the wonderful action of mental forces in the region of the subconsciousness, and how such hidden action may be influenced and directed by the outward stimuli of active drugs, or by the subtle power of the new mental energies, exerted through silent telepathic communications, or through the effective reiterations of auto-suggestions.

These same investigations are showing us that this subconsciousness is the most sensitive recorder of outer influences and is perfectly responsive to the central nervous system of the body. It must, therefore, be a vastly important fact in the health, holiness and happiness of a man's life. For whatever seriously affects it, affects the very springs of life. It is no small thing, therefore, to infuse and saturate the subconsciousness with the atmosphere and ideality of health and strength. It means a new tonic quality sent out into all the nerves of being. It means a new lease on life. Such a discovery reveals the possibility of most fascinating studies in "the abyssmal depths of personality" and reveals also the possibility of mentally infusing into that region new vitality for the regenerative and constructive forces of life. It is the recognition that mind—even subconscious mind—plays a larger part than we have sometimes imagined, in the maladies and the remedies of the medical world. We all know how an ill man is kept in that condition when he is continually told that he looks badly. Many a sick person has been made worse by the unwise comments of his friends. The Job's comforters are responsible for much aggravated distress in this world. But we all know how the encouragement of the nurse and the doctor means oftentimes as much as the medicine. We are also familiar with the value of a change of scene or a change of thought in certain nervous troubles. Oftentimes this is all that is needed to dispossess the demon of habitual depression. And the pleasurable novelty of travel, with its new acquaintances and new scenes, its absolute diversion and varied interests, is oftentimes the real purpose in the prescriptions to drink the waters of Carlsbad or try the air of the Riviera.

The subtle but scientific instillation of the suggestion and promise of health is perfectly legitimate. It replaces the lethargy of depression by a new buoyancy of spirit. It sends the current of a new vitalization tingling along the nerves.

Investigations, very numerous and thorough in scientific circles in these days, have taught us a few definite things about the subconscious self, although much is yet unknown. The few definite probabilities about the subconscious self seem to be such as follows:

1. The subconscious self seems to be a normal part of our nature. It is not morbid

or uncanny in its nature or development. It was largely unknown and unstudied until recent years. Yet what we have already learned, shows it to be one of the most interesting parts of our being.

2. It does not seem to reason, but to obey and follow. It would seem possible, therefore, that it can largely be controlled. We had not realized this until recently. It seems to be governed primarily, not by reason, but by instincts and intuitions and commands. These are given, some at birth—the natal instincts; some by unconscious training and habit from earliest infancy and all through life; and some by conscious training along the line of the great principles, and the laws of life and action.

3. It seems, as some assert, to be purer, more native, simple and elemental than our conscious self—and less allied to evil and less susceptible to it. Some investigators cite a large number of experiments to prove this proposition. It seems to them conclusive that even in hypnotic suggestion, the subconscious mind will not respond to a distinctly evil suggestion or a suggestion of crime. Upon this point, scientists still differ.

4. The subconscious self seems to have

great reserves, which can be used in emergency. For instance, a mother may have to stay up night and day with her little one. Strength is given to do it. She can keep awake for much longer intervals when necessary. Or, perhaps, a man is suddenly put under heavy responsibility, and the new demands may be wonderfully met. Webster is called upon in the Senate to reply to Hayne. He calls his powers together. He makes the greatest speech of his life. He says: "All that I had ever thought or dreamed on the subject came before me saying, 'Take me! use me!'"

5. The subconscious mind to many investigators seems to be more clearly allied to the divine Spirit in the seeming fact that it never sleeps; that it often performs its highest functions when the objective senses are in abeyance; that it is infinite in its reaches. It seems to be the shores of a boundless ocean. Some believe it is in closer contact with the Universal Spirit than reason. On the other hand, Dr. Richard C. Cabot says: "It has been stated that the subconscious life is our point of contact with God and with the spiritual world in general. It does not seem to me that there is any

clear grounds for this belief. It is not obvious from examples which I have analyzed."

Nevertheless, on this point physicians and metaphysicians may long disagree. It is a matter difficult of proof. But many of us feel that both conscious and unconscious mind is nearer to the great Central and Universal Mind than we have sometimes realized or imagined.

II. THE TRAINING OF THE HIDDEN ENERGIES

THE relation of the conscious to the subconscious mind may be crudely illustrated in this way. A great ocean steamer has its captain and pilot up above, observing and reasoning, directing the vessel. Down below are the engineer and the stokers, and also the great engines, all obeying orders. So in our life. The conscious mind is above—the captain, the pilot, observing, reasoning, directing the vessel. The subconscious mind is the engineer, the stokers and the great engines themselves, following directions and furnishing the great power.

Now the question comes, in what particular ways may the subconscious self be influenced for health? This is a vital and important consideration. We may note, however, as a preface to our answer. The reason and memory, the conscious mind, seem to act through the brain; while the unconscious mind seems to act largely, not by the brain, but through the whole body by the entire nervous system, the cerebro-spinal and sympathetic system, ganglia, glands, etc., in all the various parts of the body. This theory, if correct, would account for the very important part that unconscious mind plays in all bodily functions.

Further, we need not seek to control the subconscious mind too minutely. Many things we do better by instinct than if we stop to reason about them. It is jocularly said that if the thousand-legger once stopped to reason which foot he should put forward first, he would never move an inch. So of our own deep and instinctive life. Much of it ought not to be interfered with. Much goes on better without our thought.

Therefore, all that we can wisely do is merely to affirm great truths and inspiring ideas; to live in their high and broad vision; to make them the atmosphere of our life—and then let the subconscious self work them out as it will.

We come now to our more definite answer. We said that the subconscious self seemed to be governed primarily by instinct and intuition. But it can also be governed and controlled to a large extent by the exercise of definite methods which are now being clearly recognized by modern psychology and physiology.

One method is by the stimulus of mental suggestion when we are wide awake. This process is concentration upon a certain idea or ideas until they become dominant in the thinking and life. Mental suggestion is the process and power of a new idea to stimulate and dominate the life. That is the matter in a sentence. The process of suggestion is described and discussed in many pages and chapters in our latest psychologies—its why and wherefore and modus operandi. Suggestion has been used to a greater or less extent in all medical work from time immemorial, but is beginning to be used to-day more systematically, both in ordinary practice and in all processes of psychotherapy. It is also the secret of all the various cults of mind and faith cure.

Mental suggestion is also constantly used in daily life. We govern our children oftentimes by mental suggestion. When a mother takes her little babe and croons over it a soft lullaby with such words as "Sleep, my baby, sleep," that is mental suggestion. A child has bumped its head. Mother kisses the bump and says: "Now, it is well." And it is well very soon. A child is talking and thinking along wrong lines. The mother ingeniously suggests another more interesting subject and changes the current of the child's thoughts. That is mental suggestion. A task is to be done. It looks like hard work. But by a few words we throw an imaginary glamor around the task,—"Let's play so and so, let's make believe," and how easily the task is done! That is mental suggestion.

We use the same process to some extent with adults. The ways are a little more ingenious and mature. Not merely words, but physical objects, can give the needed suggestion. Perfumes, an ornament, a certain position in an easy chair, a comfortable church pew may be all that is needed. Wives who are wise govern their husbands by love and mental suggestion. Lawyers use it as much as argument with a jury. Salesmen use it in persuading customers. There are even business schools where they teach it as a fine art most successfully. Many ministers use it consciously or unconsciously in their work, pulpit and pastoral The most successful evangelists are those who by so-called personal magnetism can plant right mental suggestion in their hearers and thus move them to right life. Why should not the same thing be used to make better health conditions?

Systematic suggestion can be effectively used in the work of improving health. Many people are in such a condition that the thing they most need is the power of a new and stimulating idea. In many cases drugs or surgery are not required. But they do need a new outlook, a mental and spiritual stimulus. This will have its physical effect. It will stimulate and reinforce and re-energize the whole system. It will help to a better circulation, more active functions, a steadier heart, better control of nerves.

Now, this is not theory. Dr. Paul DuBois, the famous French physician, gives a remarkable list of cases in his book on "The Psychic Treatment of Nervous Disorders." More recently, in the Emmanuel Movement in Boston, along the same lines, many cures have been wrought by the simple and daily use of mental suggestion.

As we mentioned at the beginning, hypnotic suggestion is sometimes used in medical practice. So much, however, can be done by simple mental suggestion in the open, and along natural and normal lines, that this method is by far much the best for general use, leaving all other forms of suggestion to medical practice.

Mental suggestion, let me repeat, is the process and power of injecting into the mind a new and stimulating idea; and to be most helpful this must be done systematically, and under such conditions as will allow the idea to become a real part of the life, and active and dominant in it. Or to put it in a more scientific way, we may use the phraseology of an eminent medical investigator of psychic phenomena, Forel, who speaks of suggestion as a "psychic (*i. e.*, mental) or more properly, psycho-physical, reaction, in which an idea usually connected with perception becomes so intense and narrow, the mind becomes so filled with 'one idea' that this idea loses its ordinary associations with its corrective counter-ideas, breaks violently through common restrictions, and releases cerebral activities that are usually independent of it and generally, if not always, subconscious." *

In suggestion, a dominating idea is presented to the mind by someone who wills to influence. In auto-suggestion, or suggestion to oneself, the process is all from within,

* Forel—*Hypnotism and Psychotherapy.*

the idea being repeated, reiterated, emphasized, until it penetrates the subconscious mind and tends to form a new habit, and give new stimulus.

"Auto-suggestion must be persistent and systematic," says one who has had much experience. "This is well to remember in any formal attempt to use such a method of self-help. Although auto-suggestion can be used at any time, the best time is when body and mind are relaxed. Auto-suggestion made just before retiring, or on waking in the morning, when the conscious part of our mind is inactive and the way to the subconscious part is clearer, or at some hour during the day when a few minutes rest can be taken in an easy chair or on the bed, seems to be particularly effective."

As a most practical series of ideal mental suggestions, for many classes of people, a book by Henry Wood of Boston called, "Ideal Suggestion through Mental Photography," can be heartily recommended. It is a most helpful and stimulating book along this line. One need not endorse everything the author says. But the substance of it is thoroughly sound, both psychologically and physiologically. He gives practical directions for the use of mental suggestion for real help toward health, both of soul and body. Such a definite and practical system of inspiring and uplifting mental suggestion cannot help becoming a splendid reinforcement in the life. I have known many who have used this very system with excellent results.

Notice, in all this, that scientific mental suggestion is thinking *to a purpose.* It differs from ordinary suggestion, fugitive ideas of suggestion, in being systematic and continual. It is mental suggestion as a definite work and purpose.

It is also sometimes most helpful if a formula of suggestion is used, as a "creative assertion," in Dr. Cabot's phrase, to be repeated over and over again, say every hour or two hours a day for a week or two weeks. This affirmation, or it may be a prayer, is made in simple language by one who understands the matter, and varies for each case to be met.

What is one really doing when he makes a "creative assertion" to a patient, or even a patient to himself? Let Dr. Cabot answer: "He is not trying merely to state facts; he is trying to improve facts, and he is mighty sure that he can do it. He would be false to his duty, he says, if he tried to take the coldly scientific point of view, and to state precisely what he thinks is going to happen in the presence of a person already sufficiently burdened with the weight of disease. For no one knows exactly what is going to happen; and, in fact, what is going to happen depends more or less upon how much *courage* you succeed in infusing into the sufferer before you. It is not a case for looking on and describing what you see; it is a case for doing things, for wrestling with fate and scoring to win." *

This we must emphasize. The very first condition for most people, if they would maintain, restore or keep their health, is to live in a healthful mental atmosphere. This is one of the most important things we have to learn. Our thinking, our daily thinking, must be done along lines which are wholesome and aspiring and uplifting. And it must, just as far as possible, ignore and inhibit thought of disease and diseased conditions.

Besides the wide-awake mental suggestion, a further method for influencing the subconsciousness is by the stimulus of mental suggestion just before sleep. Dr. Waldstein, of

* *Psychotherapy* magazine, Vol. I., No. 2.

New York, assures us of the effectiveness of this practical method. Dr. Worcester has told of numerous cures by this method, especially in the case of little children who were relieved of stammering and many bad habits of childhood.

A third method for controlling subconscious action, is the stimulus of mental suggestion during hypnotic sleep. But this should be used only under most careful medical supervision and only in extreme cases. Many practitioners with whom hypnotism once found favor have in many instances discontinued it. In the opinion of many eminent physicians, hypnotism is coming to have a limited field of usefulness in this work. For a restricted class of cases in the hands of expert men these physicians consider it beneficial. But medical opinion seems to be swinging over to the view that in many cases results which were once supposed to be possible only through hypnotism can be obtained quite as well by waking suggestions with the co-operation of the patient, without risking any of the possible dangers attending hypnotism. Dr. DuBois has shown most strikingly the value of mental therapeutics in waking suggestion. For instance, he says: "I have shown that in this influence (persuasive or educational suggestion) exercised on the patients afflicted with the various functional troubles of the digestive apparatus or the heart, or the respiratory system, there is always an element of suggestion. To arouse in the patient the conviction of cure is the fundamental indication. It is impossible for me always to keep the patient from reaching this conviction by blind faith, but the fault, if fault there be, must be imputed to the subject. Personally I take care that my statements are rationally founded; I transmit to the patient only such convictions as are based on my psychological or physiological views. I try to make the patient follow the same paths, to explain and to make him understand as clearly as possible, the influence of mental representations on organic functions." *

In general, it may be said that the educational method is among the most valuable of all psychotherapeutic measures. "This method contemplates teaching the patient what he has, what he has not, what he seems to have, what he can do, what he cannot do, and what he simply believes he cannot do." This

* Dr. Paul DuBois—*The Psychic Treatment of Nervous Disorders.*

expresses briefly what might be much elaborated.

In the educational method, by first separating the false from the true, the real from the imaginary, the inevitable from the merely habitual, the patient becomes enlightened as to the real nature of his own case. He obtains this enlightenment "through frequent conferences with the physician, who talks to him somewhat as a physician talks to his colleague in a consultation, the method of the physician and consultant being modified in accordance with the lack of knowledge which the patient has of the anatomy and physiology necessary to a scientific understanding of the subject. The physician, so to speak, popularizes for his patient the knowledge which he possesses and which another physician would comprehend without the necessity of such popularization. Understanding his own symptoms and being led to a full belief in the possibility of their removal, the patient advances more easily along the path to recovery."

Another method of helping to control the subconscious mind is by establishing good habits. The subconscious mind seems to be largely a creature of habit. Now thought is a habit, as well as any part of our action.

If we learn to think rightly, learn to think on wholesome subjects, learn to think along the lines of health, learn to banish morbid and unwholesome subjects; in a word, if we learn to think along the lines of health, and make a habit of these things, we will wonderfully stimulate and direct the subconsciousness.

A fifth method of controlling subconscious mind for good is by the exercise of a determined will. These unconscious powers seem to respond to will-power most wonderfully. When a patient determines to be well and keep well, he will do wonders. We must not let our wills get flabby; nor be easily discouraged; nor give up after one trial, or five trials or a dozen trials. When we see the truth, we must hold steadily to it. When we map out a good course to follow, we must follow it. The subconsciousness rejoices to obey a masterly will—as much as a thoroughbred horse to obey the master.

In all these processes for the control of the subconscious self, we cannot emphasize too strongly the value of two things—concentration and repetition.

Concentration means continued and persistent thought along certain fixed ideas. Perhaps only one idea at first, but concentrate upon it—hold it steadily before the mind, look at it from different points of vision. Concentrate upon it until you absorb it—until it becomes a part of you.

In this process, repetition is also most valuable. Repeat over and over again, at stated intervals, day after day. Thus we give depth to the impression. Eternal vigilance is the price of liberty.

We must remember, in regard to this subconscious self, that we are just learning to use its powers. A hundred years ago, we had just as much electricity in earth and air as we have to-day. But we did not know how to use it. Now we do know how, and how marvelously we are using the power of electricity to-day! So with these powers of subconsciousness. We are beginning to understand and use them. We are just on the brink of further and fuller developments. But what we already know we must use in order to come to greater things.

These subconscious powers are largely latent forces. Many of us are using only a half or a third of our real equipment. We can call out the reserves of life—in these emergencies of depression or ill-health. We can release the pent-up energies for our bettering or restoration. Says Prof. James in a notable essay on "The Energies of Man": "Most of us feel as if we lived habitually with a sort of cloud weighing upon us, below our highest notch of cleverness in discernment, sureness in reasoning, or fairness in deciding. We are making use of only a small part of our possible mental and physical resources. In some persons this sense of being cut off from their rightful resources is extreme, and we get the formidable neurasthenic conditions." Prof. James goes on to show in this essay, how levels of new energy, which have long remained unutilized, may be set to work by these various methods of mental suggestion, such as we have endeavored to indicate.

Now in all this what is the chief part of religion? Much of the work of the control of the energies of the life can be done either with or without religion. But religion, by faith and prayer and by the affirmation of its great and inspiring and uplifting truths, can furnish the strongest possible stimulus in mental action. It can also supply the background of hope and assurance of the divine presence and purpose that in itself is of real benefit to both soul and body. Still further, the type of character created by true religion is the best type to resist disease—that is, the character in which the features are calmness, faith, patience, fearlessness, trustfulness, endurance, hopefulness, cheerfulness. This is the true type of true religion. This same type of character is the best resource for the restoration of health. Every one of these mental and spiritual characteristics reacts most helpfully on all the bodily functions and life.

What we must chiefly endeavor to do in all this is to make conditions of self-control more wholesome and normal. It is to come into fuller harmony with divine law—the laws both for the body and the soul. It is to come into such a spirit, by faith and prayer and obedience to truth, that our lives will eagerly welcome more of the great universal spirit of divine health and strength.

For this new life, energy, love—the power of health and happiness—is the infinite power. Its highest description is in the apostle's words: "For it is God that worketh in you, both to will and to do of His good pleasure."

FOURTH CONFERENCE

Some Elements in Morbid Moods

I. The Casting Out of Fear.
II. The Control of the Imagination.
III. The Cause and Cure of the Worry-Habit.

I. THE CASTING OUT OF FEAR.

WHAT are the morbid moods as ordinarily considered? Are they not too much self-retrospection; an over-conscientiousness; an ultra-sensitiveness, or mistrust of self, or suspicion of oneself, or of others; a sense of inferiority, or constant self-depreciation and depression; the pathological state of mind—a morbid curiosity and interest in disease and diseased condition; or a constant bondage to fear, such as fear of failure, fear of sickness, fear of death? The perpetually discouraged life is a form of morbidity. The moods of cynicism and pessimism are essentially morbid moods; for they do not look at life healthily; nor do they give out healthful influences. These, in general, are the chief forms of the morbid moods, and some of the forms at least that we consider in this address.

Morbid moods are no new ailments. The patriarch Job was in one when he was so depressed that he bewailed the day of his birth.

Elijah under the juniper tree is another instance; David, when he cried "Why art thou cast down, O my soul?"; Solomon, when he felt—"All is vanity and vexation of spirit." And the same infection has come at times to modern spirits—even to the gifted ones of earth. Let me quote from several:

Goethe says: "I will say nothing against the course of my existence. But at bottom it has been nothing but pain and burden, and I can affirm that during the whole of my seventy-five years I have not had four weeks of genuine well-being. It is but the perpetual rolling of a rock that must be raised up again forever."

Luther wrote: "I am utterly weary of life." The Electress Dowager one day when Luther was dining with her, said to him: "Doctor, I hope you may live forty years to come." "Madam," he replied, "rather than live forty years more, I would give up my chance of Paradise."

Bunyan's experience, as he wrote it, was this: "I was both a burthen and a terror to myself; nor did I ever so know as, now, what it was to be weary of my life, and yet afraid to die. How gladly would I have been anything but myself!"

Concerning one period of his life, Tolstoi wrote: "I felt that something had broken within me on which my life had always rested; that I had nothing left to hold on to, and that morally my life had stopped. . . . I did not know what I wanted. I was afraid of life. I was driven to leave it: and in spite of that I still hoped something from it. My state of mind was as if some wicked and stupid jest was being played on me by some one. One can live only so long as one is intoxicated, drunk with life; but when one grows sober, one cannot fail to see that it is all a stupid cheat. What is truest about it is that there is nothing funny or silly in it; it is cruel and stupid, purely and simply. . . . But perhaps (I often said to myself) 'there may be something I have failed to notice or to comprehend.' It is not possible that this condition of despair should be natural to mankind. And I sought for an explanation in all the branches of knowledge acquired by man. I questioned painfully and protractedly and with no idle curiosity. I sought, not with indolence, but laboriously and obstinately for days and nights together. I sought like a man who is lost and seeks to save himself—and I found nothing. I became convinced, moreover, that all those who before me had sought for an answer in the sciences have also found nothing. And not only this, but that they have recognized that the very thing which was leading me to despair—the meaningless absurdity of life—is the only incontestable knowledge accessible to man."

To those who are interested in a very detailed history and description of these moods, I would recommend Prof. James' most interesting book on "The Varieties of Religious Experience," and especially the chapters on "The Sick Soul," and "The Religion of Healthy-mindedness."

At this time, however, let us consider three chief classes of morbid moods which are especially prevalent.

The first group are the morbid moods of fear.

From childhood on, many are afflicted with morbid fears. There is a long series of morbid anticipations, as Horatio W. Dresser points out in his "Voices of Freedom," namely, "that we shall suffer certain children's diseases, diseases of middle life and of old age; the thought that we shall grow old, lose our faculties, and again become childish; while crowning all, is the fear of death. Then there is a long line of particular fears and trouble-bearing expectations, such, for example, as ideas associated with certain articles of food, the dread of the east wind, the terrors of hot weather, the aches and pains associated with cold weather, the fear of catching cold if one sits in a draught, the coming of hay-fever upon the 14th of August in the middle of the day, or some similar date, and so on, through a long list of fears, dreads, worriments, anxieties, anticipations expectations, pessimisms, morbidities, and the whole ghostly train of fateful shapes, worthy to rank with Bradley's 'unearthly ballet of bloodless categories.'

"Yet this is not all. This vast array is swelled by innumerable volunteers from daily life, the fear of accident, the possibility of calamity, the loss of property, the chance of robbery, of fire, or the outbreak of war. And it is not deemed sufficient to fear for ourselves. When a friend is taken ill, we must forthwith fear the worst and apprehend death. If one meets with sorrow . . . sympathy seems to enter into and increase the suffering."

So also Horace Fletcher says in one of his books—"Happiness as Found in Forethought,

Versus Fearthought,"—" Fear has had its uses in the evolutionary process, and seems to constitute the whole of forethought in most animals; but that it should remain any part of the mental equipment of human civilized life is an absurdity. I find that the fear element of forethought is not stimulating to those more civilized persons to whom duty and attraction are the natural motives, but is weakening and deterrent. As soon as it becomes unnecessary, fear becomes a positive deterrent, and should be entirely removed, as dead flesh is removed from living tissue."

"Man often has fear stamped upon him before his entrance into the outer world," adds Mr. Henry Wood in one of his treatises. "He is reared in fear; all his life is passed in bondage to fear of disease and death, and thus his whole mentality becomes cramped, limited, and depressed, and his body follows its shrunken pattern and specification. . . . Think of the millions of sensitive and responsible souls among our ancestors who have been under the dominion of such perpetual nightmare! Is it not surprising that health exists at all? Nothing but the boundless divine love, exuberance, and vitality, constantly poured in, even though unconsciously to us, could in some degree neutralize such an ocean of morbidity."

Now what are the causes of these morbid moods? They are various, but we may mention the principal ones. The cause of course may be physical—some organic trouble—some diseased condition, or possibly only a slight derangement. It may be climacteric condition, when the internal system of our life is undergoing a serious readjustment, such as oftenest happens at the age of puberty, or at twenty, forty or sixty years of age. Or, it may be nervous exhaustion, overwork, or over-worry, or wrong habits of life. Or bad hygiene—such as results in indigestion, a torpid liver and other derangements. Another cause may be a too delicate constitution. Some may be too sensitively built. The tough-fibered do not usually have these moods or troubles. Still another cause may be the inability to meet the real troubles of life—the actual failures, sickness and losses of property or loved ones. Or the cause may be wrong mental habits—the point of view mentally false or inadequate. Or the cause may be the unregenerate nature. The need of a new birth spiritually—a new frontage toward man, the universe and God.

What is the cure of morbid moods? I need not remind you that there is no one cure. But there are various cures, according to the nature and cause of the disease, and the treatment needed is often a combination of both physical and mental and spiritual.

Mental treatment may help to make better conditions for further work, although when an organic trouble is the cause, the initial and necessary treatment must be conducted by regular medical or surgical care. The physical trouble must be righted first of all. You all know that if the cause is nervous exhaustion, as it is in many cases, the first thing is to build up the nervous system again by rest-cure, by frequent feeding, and by psychic treatment. If the cause is climacteric condition, the best cure is to be as patient as one can—a change of scenery when possible, and as much light and wise amusement as can be given. When the cause is bad digestion, the best cure probably is to learn to eat wholesome food and to masticate thoroughly. When the cause is the liver, more outdoor exercise is needed, more fresh air. It is true that bad hygiene, bad air, and lack of exercise are responsible for many morbid moods. If the cause of the morbid moods be a delicate constitution and a sensitive nature, we must use all reasonable means to build up physical strength and to harden ultra-sensitiveness. And when wrong mental habits are the cause, there must come a re-education of the mind into right thinking and a persistent exercise of the will-power along right lines.

These directions may be suggestive and helpful. We may say to these afflicted ones: Seek cheerful society. There is nothing better than the company of little children and of cheerful, healthy people. Take up some wholesome reading—avoid all else. Read a funny paper. Keep to the cheerful side of the Bible. If the cause is lack of spiritual vision, the sense of sin and the oppression of fate, then what is needed is a new spiritual experience in the life, bringing a new vision and trust in God.

We may say, in a word, that fear is the negative and abnormal condition of the inner life. Love is the normal, the divine equipoise. The process of the casting out of fear is the process of expelling an intruder and of bringing the life again into its natural, right, and wholesome condition. It is the very law of physics: "Two bodies cannot occupy the same space at the same time." As one comes in, the other must go out. The heart at the start may be full of fear. Trust or love begins to come in. Fear is pushed out. And when the heart is full of trust, there is no place left for fear. For these are mutually exclusive. Perfect love means the heart full of love, the heart in which fear has no place.

Some of you can remember, as I do for myself, when your life was lived continually under fear. You feared ghosts and evil spirits; you feared disease; you feared failure; you dreaded God. You feared death; a thousand fears had possession of your life. But many of these fears you have conquered. It is a gradual process, but it may go on.

We can drive out fear by a new mental and spiritual outlook—a supreme confidence in God. We must say to ourselves—"We must not fear; we will not fear."

As Dr. Richard Cabot says: "What such persons need above all is to cultivate their inner resources, to strengthen their powers of defense against the discouragement, the anxiety, the depression which may flow into them as the result of whatever disagreeable or threatening events they meet. Nervous people are prone to take the color of their surroundings; they are oversensitive to the buffets and shocks of life. They need, above all, the power to resist, to shut out, to turn away from the compelling assertions of their environment, whether that environment be a commanding person, or a murky day, or a pain." *

The surgeon must be fearless; his hand must not tremble in the operation. That would be fatal. He must have confidence in himself and his work. The artist must not fear, else his trembling strokes will damage all his work. He must work only in faith and confidence in his skill.

So we in our life and work must not fear. We must go forward confidently with faith in ourselves and God. We are put here for work. No cringing, no trembling, but earnest and brave service. Perfect trust is that full, and frank communion by which we realize that the Father is with us. Perfect trust is the day's bravery in the fellowship of the divine. Perfect trust is the conquest of fear through the absorbing consciousness of God.

There is something splendid when a man walks the ways of life and does strong deeds, without the least particle of fear in his soul,

* *Psychotherapy* magazine, Vol. I., No. 1.

serene and strong in his faith in God; dauntless and deathless in his grasp on life and eternity; free and fearless in all his spiritual doings and explorations; standing up in the dignity of the spiritual manhood that God has given him.

II. THE CONTROL OF THE IMAGINATION

THE second class of morbid moods which we are to consider at this time, are the morbid moods of a diseased imagination.

Imagination is a real factor in every one of our lives. We may not have the genius of imagination, but we have imagination. We dream of the future, and imagine what will be. We are constantly using imagination. We may use it prosaically or poetically; we may use it ignobly or beautifully; we may use it wholesomely or disastrously.

Do we often enough consider this fact: the world of imagination in every one of us has its sins and its sanctities? "The sins of the imagination" is a subject not often treated and yet it is a most important and vital one. The imagination has a close relation to deeds. Every sin in the life is first committed in the imagination.

We hear of some one gone wrong. We cannot think how it happened. For that person had been well-brought up, always appeared respectable, always seemed most normal. But the secret is here. It was, in a sense, a double life. Outwardly it was moral, as far as deeds go; but inwardly, and in the imagination, it was immoral. A great tree in the forest sometimes seems perfectly sound. But a blow at its trunk pulverizes it. It is rotten within. An insect has eaten out its heart and strength. The same thing may happen in a life.

A physician recently called attention to this matter in the following words: "Books are mainly silent on the subject of the diseased imagination. Fathers and mothers shrink from talking to their children about these things. Yet an impure word, a doubtful jest, a tale of wickedness is drunk in by these children, and excites the imagination and often does untold injury. In the realm of the imagination there is an enchanted middle ground between virtue and vice in which many a soul lives and feeds in secret. To them it seems to be harmless and without the pale of actual sin. There is no intention to sin, but only to filch the pleasure of imagination. But it is a sin. The willing secret indulgence of the imagination is a gross evil, and one of the most dangerous of practices." *

There is more ignoble use of the imagination than we sometimes think or confess. Many who would scorn the actual sin, indulge their imaginations viciously; they think in the freest, most irresponsible way; they talk about things which they have no right even to think about; they read about things that are salacious and that remain in the imagination as an unwholesome and disastrous influence.

What excuses do they give themselves in these matters? They seem to consider that the world of imagination is a free world, in which they can do whatsoever they will, without law or restriction. What is imagination, they say, except something unreal and unsubstantial? Some souls, whose actual lives afford few real pleasures, think that they can indulge as they please in the pleasures of imagination.

Do we say that it is impossible to control the imagination? Perhaps it is impossible to control it absolutely; but we can hold it in check, and it is surely possible not to

* J. D. Plunket, M. D., Nashville, Ky.

stimulate and feed imagination with unwholesome nourishment.

Do any say that they have immunity in the field of imagination, since if it harms anybody, it will be nobody but themselves? But they must remember, they never harm themselves without harming others. "We are members one of another." Do we say that as long as thoughts do not issue in deeds, our thoughts are guiltless? We would scorn to do wrong; scorn to steal, scorn to murder, but yet do our thoughts circle sometimes round the whole compass of the commandments, and we think unworthy thoughts against God and man.

This is the great truth. It needs iteration and reiteration. Our thought is *real*—it is an actual and substantial part of us. Our imagination *does* count; our thought is a *deed!* It makes our life. God's word saith: "As a man thinketh in his heart, so is he."

These sins of imagination are dangerous in two ways. First they make temptation easier to us, by accustoming us to the thought of the sin. Some love to play with fire. Some love to walk along the edge of the precipice of temptation. It is most perilous; it is dallying with sin; it is inviting, even welcoming temptation. It is the first step to the overt act. Never comes the deed, unless it is first committed in the imagination.

These imaginations also actually stain and weaken the fiber of the soul. An evil suggestion makes a strong impress upon the memory. It brushes off the bloom from the soul, and almost inevitably spoils something of the nobler life. An evil and unwholesome imagination may contaminate the very springs of life. It may create a subtle poison in the atmosphere. It may make the imagination permanently diseased, and thus a chronic curse in the life.

Moreover, these vicious or unwholesome imaginations, often become in themselves actual sin. If the evil thought come suddenly, and is resisted and scorned and flouted, no harm may be done. But if it come, and is nourished and cherished, and rolled as a sweet morsel under the tongue, then real sin is committed in the soul. It is the willing harboring and indulging of unworthy and ignoble imaginations that is the fatal thing.

This subtle peril begins in the earliest years, and some phases of it are life-long. Imagination is fresh and strong in childhood and youth. Children are wonderfully full of imagination and of an insatiate curiosity, although they are at first absolutely pure-minded. There has been many a case of evil imagination in childhood made and fostered by unwholesome surroundings or companions or habits. Parents should exercise wisdom in training the children, and teaching them so that the imagination may be directed into right channels. They should give the children plenty of good reading, and fill their lives with good wholesome friends and recreations, leaving no room for the evil influences.

There is so much yellow journalism in our day which panders to a vicious and morbid imagination, there is so much in modern literature that is unsavory, so much in modern theaters and their bill-board advertisements that is vicious and depraving. There are so many low places of amusement, frequented by children and young people, which are constant incitements to vicious imagination and actual vice. These things are the real menace in our present-day life.

Parents complain that their children are getting away from them—that they are losing a taste for solid reading and serious things, and that they constantly crave excitement. In youth they are already burning the candle at both ends, living at the pace that kills, wasting their reserves, and becoming reckless and morbid in their moods.

Much of the trouble comes from the constant stimulation of imagination along unwholesome and morbid lines.

Fathers and mothers are largely responsible for these things. They ought to know what their boys and girls are reading, and what they are seeing. Perhaps a little more real companionship with their children, a little more careful and wholesome guidance, would mean much for them, and for the future years.

There comes the practical question: How can we definitely control the imagination, how can we purify our thought, how can we get rid of the morbidities and iniquities of the imagination and restore the sanctities of the inner life?

The process consists of three steps. First of all, we must have purification. We can have this only through the prayer: "Create in me a clean heart, and renew a right spirit within me." This is the beginning, the essential way. It is the work of God in the soul, purifying and renewing the life. It is the cleansing of the fountain. Nothing can come before this; nothing is so important. Other methods are palliative. This goes to the root. This is the divine work, essential and fundamental.

But the second step is also exceedingly important: preoccupation. This is our part. That is, we are to fill our mind with noble pictures and noble images. We are to read noble books, think high thoughts, keep in a wholesome atmosphere. The mind must have something to work with. It will work with either good or bad material. Let it have the best material, and only this.

The third step of the process for the control of the imagination and the restoration of the sanctities of the inner life is this: Protection. We must use insistent, eternal vigilance in keeping out evil. Some evil can be seen and fought against. Books, pictures, songs, companions that are evil and vulgar, we must be resolute against. We must avoid people and places that tear down the veils of delicacy and purity in the inner life. We must set our faces resolutely against these things. We cannot play with fire without being burned. We cannot touch pitch without being defiled.

We were speaking of these visible evils.

Invisible suggestions of evil are as thick as germs in the air. We are none of us immune, except in one way; and that is, by keeping the spiritual health in good trim. If we neglect prayer and spiritual exercise and the good food of God's word, we will grow weak and liable to disease. The spiritual health is kept up by living in the light, and close to the heart of the Master.

III. THE CAUSE AND CURE OF THE WORRY-HABIT.

THE third class of morbid moods which we have to consider are those bred by the worry-habit.

What is "worry"? We all recognize it as a mental habit and a mental condition. It may be temporary or chronic. It is fret, anxiety, undue solicitude, the habit of borrowing care or trouble, the mood of apprehension, living in past regrets, present doubts and future forebodings.

It has, as you know, various technical names in medical science. It may be hypochondria —undue solicitude and worry over one's health and a morbid attention to those things. It may be unhealthy obsession along certain insistent and compulsive lines of thought. It may be neurasthenia in one of the many forms of nervous disturbance characterized by exhaustion or irritability. It may be called a phobia, any one of the many engrossing fears without an adequate cause, that seem to afflict mankind.

Says a discriminating thinker: "Worry is not to be confounded with forethought, which is the general director of our mental forces. Forethought borrows wisdom from past failures and successes, with which to lay plans for the future. True, it considers obstacles and difficulties, as a good general should, but only as hindrances which may be overcome. Forethought progresses; worry, like a squirrel in a revolving wheel, is always at the same point. . . . Worry might be defined as thought plus apprehension, moving always in a circle." *

Another puts the matter in this way: "Worry is always one of two things; it is idiocy or insanity. You may take your choice, there is no third. Worry depresses the physical vitality, destroys courage, dims the vision of the ideal, weakens the will, stands in the way of realizing anything worth while; and the human being who hopes to accomplish anything will get worry under his feet at the earliest possible moment. Work, on the other hand, good, honest, hard work, when in right relation, builds vitality and gives increased power." †

* Bishop Samuel Fallows.
† Edward Howard Griggs.

A clever magazine writer defines it well in the words: "Worry is discounting possible future sorrows so that the individual may have present misery. Worry is the father of insomnia. Worry is the traitor in our camp that dampens our powder, weakens our aim. Under the guise of helping us to bear the present and to be ready for the future, worry multiplies enemies within our own mind to sap our strength."

What are the facts about the worry habit? We know that it is gaining among Americans. It grows easily and it becomes serious. Nervous worry is now the great American disease.

Some people worry over things that have happened; their lives are filled with vain regrets. Others worry over things that are going to happen. Some people worry over actual things; others are constantly worrying over imaginary things.

But we are awakening to the seriousness of the modern conditions of overwrought life. The steady increase of sanataria and nervous hospitals, and rest-retreats are significant signs of the times. The forming in recent years of sunshine societies, of "don't worry" circles, and "hundred year" or century clubs for rational living, show that people are realizing the need of new helps to meet the new and perilous conditions.

It is not, however, the occasional and momentary times of worrying that are so pernicious. It is the continual and persistent worrying habit that is the trouble—the chronic worrying over everything—that is the morbid mood that must be cured.

This is the prevailing disease of our modern life. There is so much of it—women who are perpetually full of anxious cares, men who are full of restless nervous haste—that it seems as if St. Martha, nervous, solicitous St. Martha, were the patron saint of modern womanhood, and as if St. Vitus, quick, jerky, restless St. Vitus, were the patron saint of the business men of to-day.

Most people who are worried, worry over trifles. Some worry over the weather, and over temperature. Others worry over a spot of dirt. Some over-scrupulous housekeepers carry their house on their back wherever they go. Here one worries if a picture does not hang straight; another worries over foods, and this one over dress. Some worry over every shooting pain they have. They are always looking at their sensations through a microscope, and seeing them a thousand times greater than they actually are. Many worry over their work, over their failures; others worry over criticism or lack of appreciation. A few worry over their spiritual condition—would there were more of these. Others worry over their financial condition. Many worry over themselves; some worry over others.

Now, as to the causes of the worry habit. Many are they and various. The cause may be physical. It may be some organic trouble (possibly a slight cause but an irritating one) for which the patient ought to consult some wise physician. It may be eye strain, producing nervous tension and irritability; or it may be teeth or throat trouble. It may be physical disturbance of the liver or stomach, often responsible for a good deal. Or the worry habit may be the result of overwork and general physical and nervous exhaustion. Again, the worry habit may be temperamental. Or, the worry habit may be the result of indulgence in a wrong mental attitude toward life. It may be carping thoughts and anxious thoughts run wild. This is doubtless the most prolific cause of the worry habit. The malady is most prevalent among thoughtful people, conscientious people, good workers, among those whom we want to save from such things for the sake of themselves and the world.

True it is that the high nervous tension of our modern life is responsible for much of the worry condition. It is a restless life that many of us live—an unnatural fever. There is so much love of excitement, so great a struggle to keep up appearances, so feverish a desire to be something that we are not, such a nervous apprehension that we will be just what we actually are. There is such a living on nerves—such an unwillingness to be quiet, serene, passive and genuine—that the modern generation seems to be discovering a thousand more nerves than its ancestors, and is putting itself into condition to be irritated by trifles and to worry a mole-hill into a mountain.

How can the worry habit be cured? How can people attain to peace of mind and a cheerful philosophy of life? So that they shall be like him of whom Wordsworth speaks, in the line—

"A man of cheerful yesterdays and confident to-morrows."

It is not sufficient to say, "Don't worry," or even to ask "Why worry?" These phases themselves may grow irritating however well intended they are; nor do many find sufficient such advice as "Eliminate worry!" We want something more tangible. Unaided resolution is not sufficient. What we want is to find the simple elements out of which worry is constructed and eliminate them. We aim to take the keen edge off worry, and finally—to cure it entirely. In this way, we shall help our health, and also make better workers, worthier citizens and more agreeable companions.

This is the encouraging fact. The worry habit can be overcome. If it is temperamental—a real inheritance—even then it can be overcome, although it will be harder work. But we must understand—one cannot summarily stop worrying and be done with it. There will have to be a re-education of the mental habits. One can learn, by persistent will-power, how automatically to dismiss worry. But it may take some time. To cure the habit, one must be patient, persistent, determined to conquer. The worry habit cannot be conquered in one treatment, nor in one week. It is usually of long and gradual growth, and it will need rigorous and persistent treatment. But it can be overcome. That is the great fact! Step by step it can be conquered until the habit has disappeared, and a new mental and spiritual atmosphere has come into the life.

This is the most vital and important part of the cure, and we put it into this single sentence: *Replace the worrying thought by some other thought that will keenly interest and stimulate the life.* This is the substitute cure. It can be made effective by persistent will. It can cure. It is capable of wonderful results.

This is what it means. Deliberately choose some thought, some interest, directly opposite to that which is worrying, and interesting enough to engross attention for a time, and then concentrate attention by will power upon it. Dwell on it. Get absorbed in it. Keep steadfastly away from the worry-thought. Do not allow yourself to come back to it. Think away from it. You can do it, if you try.

This is the substance of Horace Fletcher's popular pamphlets on "Menticulture" in its different phases. This is the chief method used by Dr. Walton of Boston, in his timely and suggestive little book called, "Why Worry?"

So also Dr. Achorn says in explaining this substitute cure: "The mind can be discharged from the consideration of any vexatious subject and the attention given to the enjoyment of any other. Mind cure is simply the acquiring of control over impulses, emotions, or habits that demoralize. It substitutes other habits, if necessary. The person gains mental poise, and leans toward optimism. The mind liberates the nervous mechanism and vital fluids of the body so that all the functions, both physical and mental, are performed normally. Whether the condition recognized as a chronic disorder or disease is due to mental or physical causes, one cannot always easily determine. If the person suffering is willing to cultivate one or two new habits for the old ones he suspects, although he may not be able to see that they are the cause of his trouble, he will often be surprised at the outcome." *

This definite method, simple as it is, rests on sound psychology and physiology. The greatest things after all are often the simplest, and commend themselves to our common-sense. Psychology teaches us that obsession (and worry is a form of obsession) can only be cured by replacement. The ability to forget, to inhibit one thing and to sub-

* J. Warren Achorn, M. D., in *Religion and Medicine.*

stitute another, is one of our finest mental abilities. Physiology also shows us conclusively that we stimulate whatever we resolutely fix our attention upon. If we think unduly about our ills, our health is affected. If we forget them we get along better. Chronic introspection is a disease. Worry causes a disturbance and derangement of the entire vital system.

Let us remember, therefore: The best cure for worry is substitution. Replace the worry thought by a better thought. Choose a wholesome, stimulating thought and keep to it. Deliberately do this, and use your will-power to inforce it.

Whether there is a microbe of worry we do not know. Perhaps some enterprising doctor will discover one after awhile, and teach us also its antidote. But we do know that worry is singularly contagious and infectious. Just one person in a household with a bad case of worry is enough to demoralize the whole house, to put everybody on edge and to cast a gloom over the atmosphere of the entire family.

But the microbe of worry, whether it is in the blood or the nerves, the heart, or the soul, or the air, can often be successfully fought and conquered by a persistent will, working along the lines of substitution. Will is a marvelous antidote for a great many things, but in this matter of the worry-habit it often works almost a miracle.

Does this one method seem too general a direction? Here then, are some minor but definite matters which will help in accomplishing the substitution cure, and persons afflicted with the worry-habit might well be advised in such lines as these:

1. First, keep your physical system in tone. For, in all this work, the physical and mental must act together and help each other. Look well after your daily hygiene. If possible, take a sponge bath every morning, not necessarily cold, but with the chill just taken off. Then a rub-down with a rough towel, and a few exercises and a few minutes of deep breathing. Not too much clothing, day or night; heavy clothing irritates. A walk at least of two miles daily in the open air,—perhaps to and from the office, or better, in the country.

Arrange your life so that you can have a little vacation every day. The best time for a vacation is a little every day, and for a long vacation, just before, and not after you are exhausted. Eat regularly, slowly and masticate thoroughly. Get your hours of sleep or rest. These things will help in keeping you in fine physical trim and tone.

2. Neglect your sensations and stop that habit of introspection. Leave your mind alone, your morals alone, your conscience alone. You have paid enough attention to them. Leave your body at peace for a while. A little neglect of your internal organs will be wholesome for them and for you. You stir them up too much by thinking about them. Direct your attention voluntarily away from yourself. Get up and do something. Go out and see something. Your trouble may not be so much nervous as misdirected energy and acquiescence in inertia and despondency.

3. Take up a fad. We need diversity of interests. Fads are blessings in disguise. Take up something in which you are interested and devote some time and thought to it, even if only half an hour a day. You will think of it oftener. Photography, astronomy, music, history, old books, old prints, old furniture, a foreign language, collecting coins, studying birds or trees, pictures, golf, tennis or other things; carpenter work, wood carving, cabinetmaking, would

be good fads. One of the best is working in a garden. Such side pursuits give an interest to life, and should be encouraged.

4. Another point—pin your worries down to definite facts. Most of your worries are vague and indefinite. Many of them are imaginary. Write down in black and white what you are worrying about, and oftentimes you will see how absurd it is. The process of putting it down will clarify your vision. Sometimes at night, if you worry, promise yourself to clear it up in the morning; often that will be sufficient.

5. Learn to see the humor of the situation. Parents were worrying over their little child one night, who was fretting as they do sometimes. The situation was growing tense when the wife said—"Aren't you thankful that we do not live in the polar regions where the nights are six months long?"

A Chinese philosopher wrote ages ago: "The legs of the stork are long, the legs of the duck are short: you cannot make the legs of the stork short, neither can you make the legs of the duck long. Why worry?"

6. Be philosophical. When you miss a car, do not say, "There goes my car!" but

rather, "The next car is mine!" When you miss an engagement now and then, after trying hard to meet it, why worry over it? Such things happen to everyone now and then. Such is life. When you are traveling, do not worry because the train does not go faster, or think continually of the journey's end. Enjoy things as you go along. The speed of the train and arrival are not as vital as you think. It is vital to enjoy life now. If you fret about the weather it is futile. It will not change for you. Better make friends with the weather in all its moods. Learn to enjoy it in all its phases. Someone says: "Anyone can stand what he likes: it takes a philosopher to stand what he does not like." It is said that Canon Beadon, who lived to be very old, told a friend that the secret of long life in his own case was that he never thought of anything unpleasant after ten o'clock at night.

"You may learn," as Dr. William Osler says, "to consume your own smoke. The atmosphere is darkened by the murmurings and whimperings of men and women over the non-essentials, the trifles that are inevitably incident to the hurly-burly of the day's routine. Things cannot always go your way.

Learn to accept in silence the minor aggravations, cultivate the gift of taciturnity, and consume your own smoke with an extra draught of hard work, so that those about you may not be annoyed with the dust and soot of your complaints."

7. Live only one day at a time. You need not live your whole past through every day. You need not borrow the future years. Live this one day. It is enough. And sometimes more than enough. But we can at least get through one day bravely. Michael Angelo used to say—"To-day I endure." Prof. Palmer put it: "We can always stand it for twenty-four hours." President Lincoln had his favorite phrase for trouble: "And this too will pass." There is a quaint proverb that has a great deal of wisdom in it. It runs: "Never trouble trouble, till trouble troubles you." A certain father on his death-bed said to his children: "My children, don't worry: I have had many heavy troubles in my life, but most of them have been imaginary ones. Don't worry. It doesn't pay. Don't cross the bridge till you come to it."

But now we come to the third and most vital point—the spiritual factor in the cure of the worry habit.

Worry is no more amenable to mere physical treatment, than swearing or drunkenness. But in the treatment for a real cure must come both physical, mental and spiritual elements. We have considered the physical treatment and the mental. We have yet a few words to say about the spiritual treatment of the worry-habit.

Dr. Saleeby has pointed out that the two greatest religions the world has ever seen, Buddhism and Christianity, are essentially anti-worrying religions, though reaching the goal by very different routes. Buddhism says, "Worry is an inevitable accompaniment of life. In order to get rid of it you must destroy the desire to live, and the goal of all being is Nirvana. It means absolute acquiescence; the end of worry, because the end of life." Christianity, on the contrary says, "The great need is not less, but more abundant life. Worry is something that may be transcended, and the power by which you transcend it is trust in God and the service of man."

Another confirmation is the witness of one of our leading psychologists, Professor James, who says, "The sovereign cure for worry is religious faith. The turbulent billows of the fretful surface leave the deep parts of the ocean undisturbed, and to him who has a hold of vaster and more permanent realities, the hourly vicissitudes of his personal destiny seem relatively insignificant things." *

It is still the substitution cure that we advocate, even by spiritual treatment. Replace your doubting, restless, distrustful, faithless attitude to God, by a trustful and confident faith in God. Take God at His word. Accept and believe His promises and your worries will gradually disappear, and all life will become new.

There is one cause of worry in many lives which might well be considered in connection with spiritual treatment, and that is the fact of actual transgression in the life. This is a rightful and sufficient cause for worrying. A man should not expect peace if he lives in deliberate sin. Conscience will torment him and it ought to. Such an one is never really happy. He may seem so outwardly, but down deep in his heart there is a root of bitterness. Sin cannot be happy. The pleasures of sin have in them the sting of remorse. Anybody living in sin ought to worry and worry a great deal. For the life is wrong.

* *Talks with Teachers on Psychology.*

But such ought to do more than worry. They ought to put themselves right. There is help for them if they will, and a better life—a clean leaf for beginning a new record, and a new strength for the new life.

And yet, even among religious people we oftentimes find worry, and here it is often a want of faith in the heart. This is a very real and widely prevalent cause.

Why not trust God? Why not take Him at His word? Why not believe Him when He says that He is with us and that "all things work together for good?"

It is not unfair to say that persistent worrying is persistent unbelief—it is a subtle form of atheism. We may not intend it to be so, but so it is in its practical effects. A worrying Christian is a poor product of Christian faith—where does the faith come in at all? A Christian has no right to worry. It is doubting God's care and goodness. John Wesley used to say, "I would as soon curse and steal as worry. It is doubting God."

Learn to look on the bright side, on the divine side. Cultivate the habit. Here is a practical way of doing it. Have one of your visiting cards with such words as these written on the back—"God is love.—Count your mercies.—Worry never does any good.—Things might be worse.—All things work together for good.—Be of good cheer, says Christ.—Have faith in God." Whenever you are disposed to worry, take this card and read it, and it will change the current of your thoughts. Use this card faithfully for a while and soon you will not need it.

Napoleon, it is said, owed much of his energy, daring, prowess and success to his belief that he bore a charmed life, that he might do and dare anything, that disaster and death could not overtake him until his fate was accomplished.

But we have a deeper and truer assurance. We are in God's hands, and nothing can really or permanently harm us and there is no death for us. "All things work together for good." We can absolutetly rest in the assurance, if we will, that it is not our duty to worry about ourselves or the universe. We are not responsible for the universe. It is God's doing and He is working out His plans. So with our lives. They are God's creation and He is working out His plan in them. All that we have to do is to try our best to work with Him. Take no anxious thought for the morrow, but take thought of God.

We must remember that we cannot grow in stature by straining ourselves upward, by taking anxious thought, nor can we grow in soul by strain, introspection and agonizing. We can only grow in nature or grace by putting ourselves in the natural ways of growth, by getting into the rhythmic mood of Nature, into the deeper ways of the spirit, into fuller and fuller harmony with God's will as it is revealed to us.

We will find a deeper and richer spiritual experience as we learn to meditate often on the greatest facts of spiritual life, and come more continually to realize them in our lives. Such a habit cannot fail to bring a more joyous and confident mind and spirit, and re-act most helpfully and hopefully on the whole life, spiritually, mentally, even physically.

Such a trust and faith means resting, absolutely resting the heart continually in the promises of God. It is taking God at His word. And His word is an impregnable rock. It is like a great Gibraltar in the midst of the changing sea of human life. Times may change, friends may change, all things change, but the Gibraltar of God—a stronghold and fortress—standeth forever. We plant our feet upon the Rock of God's word. We may tremble at times. But the Rock beneath is strong as adamant, and immovable as the everlasting hills.

These are some of the mental and spiritual factors in the cure of the morbid moods of persistent fears, and of diseased imagination, and of the chronic worry-habit. Of course, they are merely suggestions of rational persuasion along these lines. Each case is a separate experiment, and the special ways of reasoning, and the mental and spiritual stimulus to be suggested, must be dictated by the circumstances involved, but in something of this method of giving a new outlook on life, may come, in many cases, the very help that is needed.

FIFTH CONFERENCE

The Higher Factors in the Re-education of the Nerves

I. The Gospel of Relaxation.
II. Work as a Factor in Health.
III. The Inspiration of the Mental Outlook.

I. THE GOSPEL OF RELAXATION

AS we have previously said, we must remember that nervous diseases are real diseases, just as real as a fever or a broken bone. They are not imaginary; they cannot be laughed away. We must comprehend the actual conditions. We must sincerely sympathize with the sufferers. But we must also be firm and confident in meeting such conditions, for in these new days nervous diseases can be treated effectively and successfully.

The first and wisest thing in any case of neurasthenia is for the patient to consult a good physician who is a specialist along these lines—and who is sympathetic to new thought and methods, and who is broad enough and wise enough to use psychology when necessary; then to follow his advice as faithfully as possible.

You know, of course, about the rest-cure, technically so-called, as used by Dr. Weir Mitchell, Dr. Playfair, Dr. Paul DuBois, and others, for twenty or thirty years past—the usual features being, first, complete rest in bed for a term of weeks; secondly, complete isolation, without letters or visits, although this has been modified in later years; and thirdly, overfeeding as frequently as possible to give increase of bodily weight. But Dr. DuBois tells us that his experience completely demonstrated that this course of treatment was rarely sufficient in itself. He found that the most effective factor in it all was the moral factor, and therefore, in all cases he advises constant use of rational psychotherapy, which he illustrates very definitely and fascinatingly in his record of twenty years' experience as given in his book "The Psychic Treatment of Nervous Disorders."

Do we know as much as we ought of that rest-cure which consists in teaching how to meet life by the doctrine of non-resistance? This is worth keeping to the fore in rational psychotherapy.

First of all, therefore, let us consider the philosophy of the rest-cure, and the new gospel of relaxation. There is much in daily life, especially with nervousness, that can be accomplished by accepting the doctrine of non-resistance a little more fully. It is a preliminary step for healing many of the ills that flesh is heir to.

Some of you perchance have read that suggestive book by Annie Payson Call, entitled, "Power through Repose," and her other book, "The Freedom of Life." These books have many chapters on this doctrine of the passive mood. They preach a veritable gospel of relaxation. Some things in the books may not perchance appeal to all of us, but yet there is plenty of good suggestion and an inspiring spirit.

Certain people work and quickly become fatigued. What is the trouble? Not the work, but the way they work. They attack their work with too much nervous tension and strain. They ought not to get fagged out by work, only wholesomely tired. When we get fatigued, we are working with too much tension at the back of the neck. We had better learn the art of the passive mood in work, that we may do the task easily and make even drudgery a pleasure. We had better get a new attitude to our work.

Many people sleep and get no rest. They have the resistance habit. They are almost as tired in the morning as when they went to rest. Perhaps they sleep in a cramped position, all doubled up, or with insufficient ventilation, or without relaxing the mind. They work all night in their sleep, if they sleep at all. They had better learn the passive mood. It can cure all this.

Many people eat regularly, three times a day—in an attitude of resistance to life. They do not get the full benefit of their food. They eat too much, or not enough, or too fast, under a strain and tension. They had better relax mind and body, eat slowly and in the attitude of the passive mood. They will find better digestion.

Some people allow even their amusements to wear them out—all strain, tension, excitement, emotions rampant, nerves on the stretch. They had better learn the art of relaxation and make amusements a real recreation.

There are those who let their sympathies wear them out in resisting the sorrows of suffering and calamity. Such sympathy is weak and sentimental. A true, large sympathy is strengthening. They need to get their sympathies on a higher plane, where they can relax in the larger vision of the blessing that suffering and calamity may bring.

A man has some hard problem to solve.

He gets into a highly wrought nervous condition over it, and it becomes more and more difficult and no nearer solution. In despair he leaves it; he relaxes; he goes about something else. And when after a time he comes back, the problem seems to solve itself. In reality, it is because he has allowed subconsciousness to work, and also has come back to it with clearer brain and rested nerves.

Many mothers wear themselves out resisting their children. Their whole idea of training seems to be resistance. They had better learn the art of acceptance and guidance. All vehemence is weak; all nagging is wrong.

Some patients are constantly resisting. The doctor has to say—"Now just relax. Just be passive and let Nature have a chance to do her work. Don't worry about the office. Make up your mind to take a rest while you are here. Don't resist. Accept. And you will get well twice as soon."

What does all this mean? Does it not indicate that we ought to use and to teach the doctrine of the passive mood a great deal more than we do? We are too much on the strain, on high tension in life. We get into the chronic condition of excited nerves, of muscles contracted, taunt, tense, and we forget how to relax.

We get so into the habit of persistent resistance that we wear ourselves out. The habit of resistance is at the root of worry, hurry, strain and irritability. Continual mental resistance gives brain fag; continual physical resistance gives nervous exhaustion.

Therefore, it is a part of wisdom to learn to relax mind and body. The gospel of relaxation has a great lesson for daily life, even on the physical side. Notice people on the street. Most of them are sad looking. They are absorbed, intent on themselves or their troubles. Look at people in a street car. Most of them have a drawn look in their features—faces grown hard with the constant habit of resistance against the world, and feeling that the world is against them. Chronic resistance has become fixed habit. It is all wrong.

All methods of mental healing inculcate the value of passivity in their treatment. The first thing is to place the patient in a comfortable position in an easy chair, and to command him: "Relax, now, relax every muscle! Be as passive as you can." This is the necessary condition before help can be given. It is a complete surrender. It is giving up to a higher wisdom for a time. But relaxation is not an end in itself. It is only a preliminary condition to something better—something positive, stimulating, and inspiring, and that something better is the strengthening and helpful truth persistently affirmed and reaffirmed in right mental suggestion.

Moreover, the doctrine of the passive mood has its wisdom on the moral side, and this will also help in controlling the nerves. As an attitude to life, it is the triumphant way. If we are continually resisting and worrying over circumstances, life is a hard fight. But if we are willing to fail, willing to be poor, willing to suffer if needs be, willing to die when our time comes—as Stevenson says,

> "Glad have I lived and glad will I die,
> And I lay me down with a will,"—

then we have lost the fear of all these things and can live life comfortably and bravely. If we realize that life's circumstances, whatever they may be, are not limitations or punishments, but opportunities for a nobler triumph, then will come the power of new conquest in life.

As a method of meeting antagonists in the ordinary ways of life, the passive mood has its advantages. When a man shows fight, it stirs up fight. Resistance excites counter-resistance. Force arouses all the antagonism. Systematic opposition, even to a child, develops all the wrong nature in him. When you meet a blatant fighter, he does not impress you nearly so much as one who does not fight at all, but just holds the truth strongly and asserts it calmly.

There is a modern as well as ancient wisdom in the words—"A soft answer turneth away wrath; but grievous words stir up anger." When we allow ourselves to lose our temper, we always lose more than we gain. When we cultivate the fighting spirit, we are arousing the passions in us which secrete a poison in our system, and disorder all our inner life. The spirit of calmness; the taking of insult, or even of injustice, with equanimity is an attitude worth cultivating.

The Japanese art of self-defense called Jiu-jutsu is a most suggestive illustration as Lafcadio Hearn explains it. Jiu-jutsu means literally conquering by yielding, and this is really the essential feature of the defense. It looks something like wrestling to our modern eyes, but the fine art of it is the gentle art of non-resistance. The purpose is to encourage the antagonist to deal his heaviest blows and gracefully escape them. So skillfully is it learned and practiced that, in his defense, an adept can make one who is unskillful unloose a joint or break his arm by a mere wrench at a vulnerable point. The stronger the opponent the worse his discomfiture. It is intelligence and skill against brute force. This is all suggestive.

In the physical way and for psychical healing, the doctrine of the passive mood is a preliminary to the further work. It is a clearing away of the barriers. It is making the right conditions for a positive work. It is the attitude of receiving. And that work, as we said, is largely the instilling into the passive mind and into the subconsciousness of the relaxed muscles, the positive affirmations of truth, of purity, of health, of the divine life.

II. WORK AS A FACTOR IN HEALTH

THESE few suggestions as to the value of relaxation, and especially as it is carried out under careful direction in a rest-cure, lead us to consider a further step in the re-education of the nerves—and that is the work-cure.

It is healthful to work. But it must be reasonable work to be healthful. A most excellent rule for the division of the day is the ancient one, ascribed to Alfred the Great: —"Eight hours for work, eight hours for play, eight hours for sleep." That seems natural and sensible. None of us should do more than eight good hours of hard work and even less, if it is continuous intellectual work. Eight hours of play means the time for meals, recreation and social life. Every life should have some recreation every day. And then eight hours for sleep—genuine sleep or at least the absolute rest in the quiet. Now it is an exceptional individual who can do with less than this amount of rest. It is not wise to cut off any of these hours of rest. It is suicidal to burn the candle at both ends.

The old but divine command: "Six days for work, but the seventh day is the Sabbath of the Lord your God," must not be forgotten. One day in seven is not yours; it belongs to God. God would make it for you a day of real refreshment of soul and body—no physical labor; none of the occupations of the week—no blanket newspapers, full of secular matter; but a new day—a day of opportunity, a day of new vision; a time of worship with God in the sanctuary; a new glimpse into God's Word; a walk in the fields with God; a visit of kindness or sympathy to some of God's children; a day of divine rest and recreation and love.

Many people are spoiling their lives by making all seven days alike. They break the divine law. Some devote six days to selfish competition and the seventh day brings no vision—how can such people see life as it ought to be, or do their work with any heart? Six days devoted to hard and reasonable work and the seventh day devoted to the things of the higher life—will make work a blessing and a health in the life.

Now work is not merely a necessary factor in every day's good health—a part of the natural law for the preservation of health—but work may also become a means of restoration to health.

The value of enjoyment on the physical side gained by self-forgetful work is well brought out by Forel, in his "Hygiene of Nerves and Mind." He says: "We must banish pleasure-seeking (but not pleasure itself) from our lives. Every pleasure cultivated for its own sake leads to ennui and disgust and injures the nervous health. Every healthy enjoyment must be earned by an harmonious mode of life. It is a pleasure to sleep, even on a hard bench, if you are tired; or to eat crude dishes, if you are hungry. To drink pure water is a healthy enjoyment, if you have a natural thirst, and it does not injure one like the satisfaction of the artificial thirst for alcohol that results in poisoning. Mental work is a healthy pleasure, if the need for muscular exercise and activity beside it is also satisfied. Muscular work is a pleasure when alternated with activity of thought and feeling, but not when carried on purely mechanically and automatically without any active attention;

for then it does not replace either abstract thought or emotional excitement, which can both be present to lead us astray in spite of such work."

There may be a very interesting comparison instituted between Omar Khayyám and Ecclesiastes. Both emphasize this present life; both seem rather pessimistic; both say—"do your best to enjoy life." But how different are the ways that they suggest.

Omar's ideal of enjoyment is:

"A Book of Verses underneath the Bough,
A Jug of Wine, a Loaf of Bread—and Thou
Beside me singing in the Wilderness—
O Wilderness were Paradise enow!"

It is careless, easy, lazy ideal. The useless life expressed in the Italian—"dolce far niente"—the sweet pleasure of doing nothing.

But in Ecclesiastes the ideal of enjoyment is this, thrice repeated and emphasized as the keynote of the book: "I know that there is no good but for a man to rejoice, and to do good in his life . . . and to enjoy the good of all his labor, it is the gift of God."

Again: "There is nothing better for a

man than that . . . he should make his soul enjoy good in his labor. This also I saw that it was from the hand of God."

And still again: "Wherefore I perceive that there is nothing better than that a man should rejoice in his own works; for that is his portion." That is, it is the life of usefulness that is the best life and the happiest.

In a word, this is the difference between Omar Khayyám and Ecclesiastes. Omar's chief figure is an idler, a loafer, a dilettante. But Ecclesiastes' is a worker, rejoicing in his work, loving his work and enjoying it, full of practical thrift and wholesome service.

However the present popularity of Omar Khayyám is a sign of reaction against absorption in theological subtleties and speculations. It is real appreciation of this life. Its attractive theme is—"Let's make the most out of this life."

But this is also the equally attractive theme of Ecclesiastes, treated in a much wiser way. Ecclesiastes is a much greater book. It is not morbid, but wholesome, when looked at rightly. It is not melancholy, but inspiring. It is an exposition of the best that was then known. Its chief theme is, Do not worry about the future, but work in the present with all your strength, and it will be your joy!

It is not work that kills, not even hard work. We may work hard every day until we are physically tired, but if we have good food and sufficient sleep, we may be able to stand it for a long stretch. But put hard work and worry together and there the mischief is done. It is not hard work, but worry that kills. We have instances of this every day.

"This world," as one says truly, "was given us to work in and to play in. It is a pretty place; but thousands of people under existing conditions seem to make a nightmare out of ordinary work and living. . . . Under the stress of modern competition one-half of mankind overpowers the other half and then has them to take care of as invalids. Women compete with men under the laws made for men, although women are rated half as strong physically as men." All these things make hard working conditions.

It is most pitiable to see many people, who know better, wearing themselves out even in social settlements and philanthropic work because they will not stop a minute. Some excellent school teachers are on the strain from one week's end to another and at the end of the term are nervous and physical wrecks. One splendid teacher, however, told me once when I asked her how she kept in such exceptional and prime physical condition, "I take a little vacation every day and I do not worry." She was a fine worker, a hard worker, but she did not worry.

Oh for the gift of knowing when to stop work! Work does become fascinating and absorbing. We think we must do it; or we have the passion for finishing it. We say, "just an hour or two more and it is finished." We work even when the warning has been given, and we know we should not continue.

This I contend. We know when we ought to stop. The instinct, God-given, is within. Often it has been emphasized in our lives by bitter and costly experience. If we are sensible, we will obey the inherent laws of God, live in a cheery wholesome mental atmosphere and use our common sense and we can do good work and full work.

For many people, work is salvation—the occupation-cure is the very thing that is needed. Some people are afflicted with worry, nervous fears, abnormal restlessness or melancholia; and then, oftentimes, the very best thing is to get them to do something; to get them interested in work, thus taking their thoughts as far as possible from themselves and their condition. Many sanitariums use these methods very effectively.

It is thoroughly proved by many experiences. Physical exercises requiring fixed attention often exert a most beneficial influence on certain classes of nervous sufferers. Such pleasant work as cataloging, clay-modeling, gymnastic exercises are frequently of the greatest value.

Most of us know that it is a great deal more tiresome to have nothing to do than to be full of work. The happiest people in this world are not the idlers; they are those who are busy all the time, those who work and work hard. If work was ever a curse, now it is a blessing. It is only when it becomes overwork that it is a curse.

Do you remember that paragraph in Lecky's "Map of Life?" He is quoting from a famous physician, Dr. Mortimer Granville: "The best way to live well, is to work well. Good work is the daily test and safeguard of personal health. . . . The practical aim should be to live an orderly and natural life. We were not intended to pick our way through the world, trembling at every step. . . . It is worse than vain, for it encourages and increases the evil it attempts to relieve. . . . I firmly believe," he continues, "that one-half of the confirmed invalids of the day could be cured of their maladies if they were compelled to live busy and active lives and had no time to fret over their miseries. . . . One of the most seductive and mischievous of errors in self-management is the practice of giving way to inertia, weakness and depression. . . . Those who desire to live should settle this well in their minds, that nerve power is the force of life and that the will has a wondrously strong and direct influence over the body and nervous system."

But another helpful thought we would emphasize—not only is work a part of the divine law of our being for possessing health; not only is work often the best means for the restoration of health—but this thought: We ought to have as a constant mental background and spiritual stimulus the conviction that God has given us work to become the greatest joy of our lives.

We must realize that when we work, we are working with Him. We must rejoice in our work, because in doing it, we are in fellowship with the divine creative power. Here we come to the most inspirational and tonic part of the philosophy of work. We need this spiritual stimulus. We are to rejoice in our work, for it is a blessing to humanity. The world needs all kinds of workers. Hand workers are just as much needed as brain workers. The farmer in the field is just as much needed as the statesman in the cabinet.

Go into a carpenter's shop. The song of the plane takes one back to the carpenter shop at Nazareth. Go into a great machine shop and see them working in the solid iron and steel, and see the great machines running so majestically, unerringly, inevitably in their work. Such a visit puts tonic into our blood. What an interesting place is one of our great merchant stores! A great hive of industry, where each has his special field!

Stand in a colossal city like New York, and wonder how such an immense city with its millions would ever find its food—a million loaves of bread every day, rivers of milk, a hundred head of cattle every day. But the problem is solved by that unique law of supply and demand, and the busy activities of thousands and tens of thousands of workers, each doing his useful part.

The whole world is as busy as a bee. Upon this incessant toil of the multitudes depends the life and happiness of existence. Each one fits somewhere, each one has his niche in the order of existence, each one must bring his contribution toward the general welfare. Whatever our work may be, by brain or hand, humble or conspicuous, at home or in public, whatever it is, if it be honest work, it is a blessing to humanity, and if we do it faithfully, we are benefactors of the race.

Blessed is that man who sees deeply into his work. There is no work but what is pleasurable, and intensely interesting, if the worker takes the trouble to get below the surface of his task. The strength and variety of materials, the miracle of natural action, the marvel of mechanics, the dexterity or ingenuity of hand or mind, the possibilities of improvement, the satisfaction of achievement—these are all full of an ever-growing interest and surprise, to one who sees deeply. If our work is commonplace or tedious in our chosen field or profession, depend upon it, it is because we ourselves are growing commonplace or tedious.

No honest work ought to be beneath us. No useful or beautiful thing is unworthy of our best efforts in the making. There is nothing in Nature, however trifling or obscure, but the divine wisdom and strength wrought in its making. God's work is not merely religious work. We have strange notions, and limit God's work most curiously. God's work is also material work—physical and artistic. Everything that man has done, God has done before him. Every invention of man, God had previously invented in His brain. So all good work is work with God. Deuteronomy says expressly—"Say not in thine heart, my power and the might of my hand hath gotten me this wealth. But thou shalt remember the Lord, thy God; for it is He that giveth thee power to get wealth." It is also said expressly that all artificers of the temple worked under the inspiration of the Almighty.

The inspiration of the Almighty! What is the ultimate purpose of this man's making shoes, and that one selling grain, and that one doing farming, and the other weaving shawls? Is it to the end of physical wealth or comfort? Mark you! The purpose of all work is that we may enter into true life, and feel sympathy with the divine purpose. In a word, it is to enter into closer fellowship with the divine. Work ought not to be a mere bread and butter strife, not a mere pot-boiling business. It is a divine fellowship in the art of a divine creation. All work and all labor are hints of God's continual work. Every work is, to a greater or less extent, a similitude of the work of creation. It is a transformation by will power and intelligence of forces and materials. This is the mental attitude that can make work a joy, a strength and an inspiring factor of health. We must learn to see the divine quality of work. Such a view of work as this, if we can bring it home to those who most need it, will be a real help in making work interesting, and will be profitable in the re-education of the nerves.

III. THE INSPIRATION OF THE MENTAL OUTLOOK

WE come more definitely to the mind-cure in this same process of restoration of the nerves to equilibrium. And the first question which confronts us is, Can the nerves be helped by a larger and truer mental outlook?

For the slighter degrees of nervous exhaustion, and especially for the preservation of our nervous system in good health, some of the following mental and spiritual suggestions may prove helpful to many. They are founded on sound psychology and physiology, although they may seem simplicity itself.

1. We do not begin to value at its full worth such a mental factor as cheerfulness, both in the maintenance of health and the cure of the slighter forms of nerve disorders.

Here is the testimony of a physician: "In the maintenance of health and the cure of disease, cheerfulness is a most important factor. Its power to do good like a medicine is not an artificial stimulation of the tissues to be followed by reaction and greater waste, as is the case with many drugs; but the effect of cheerfulness is an actual life-giving influence through a normal channel, the results of which reach every part of the system. It brightens the eye, makes ruddy the countenance, brings elasticity to the step, and promotes all the inner force by which life is sustained. The blood circulates more freely, the oxygen comes to its home in the tissues, health is promoted and disease is banished." *

Nor is it all merely therapeutic. Cheerfulness has its practical everyday value in the business world. "A sunny, cheerful, gracious soul," as one says, "is like an ocean breeze in sultry August, like the coming of a vacation. We welcome it because it gives us at least temporary relief from the strenuous strain of life. Country store-keepers look forward for months to the visits of jolly, breezy traveling men, and their wholesale houses profit by their good-nature. Cheerful-faced and pleasant-voiced clerks can sell more goods and attract more customers than disagreeable ones. Promoters, organizers of great enterprises, must make a

* Dr. A. J. Sanderson.

business of being agreeable, of harmonizing hostile interests, of winning men's good opinion. Newspaper men, likewise, depend on making friends to gain entrée, to get interviews, to discover facts, and to find news. All doors fly open to the sunny man, and he is invited to enter, when the disagreeable, sarcastic, gloomy man has to break open the door to force his way in. Many a business success is founded on courtesy, cheerfulness and good humor." *

2. Besides cheerfulness, there is real worth in the cultivation of courage. Courage is a mental condition that can be cultivated and it is of distinct therapeutic value.

So Dr. Marden, editor of the "Success" Magazine writes: "If young people only knew the power of affirmation, of the habit of holding in the mind persistently and affirming that they are what they wish to be, that they can do what they attempt, it would revolutionize their whole lives, it would exempt them from most of their ills and troubles, and carry them to heights of which they scarcely dream."

3. A serene and sunshiny life is food and tonic for the nerves. It is no small or un-

* Dr. Marden in *Every Man a King.*

important task to cultivate sunshine in the life. A sunny serene outlook makes better work.

Recall the mental balance and equipoise of spirit in the great poets, such as Shakespeare, Tennyson and Browning. They are serene and optimistic, because of their large vision. Undoubtedly it is true, as one says: "The work turned out by a calm balanced mind is healthy and strong. There is a vigor and naturalness about it that is not found in the work done by a one-sided man, a mind out of balance. Serenity never dwells with discontent, with anxiety, with over-ambition. It never lives with the guilty, but dwells only with a clear conscience; it is never found apart from honesty and square dealing, or with the idle or vicious."

4. Good sleep is food and strength to the nerves and a serene and sunny mental outlook gives better sleep. One physician says: "I know a few people who have learned the supreme art of preparing for a sweet, peaceful, restful, refreshing sleep by reversing the brain processes which have perplexed them and bothered them during the day. They have learned the secret of shutting out all their troubles, trials and perplexities, of lock-

ing them in the store or office or factory when they turn the key at night. They never drag their business troubles home. They consider themselves at play from the moment they leave work until they get back again. Nothing can induce them to be bothered or bored with anything relating to business. They have learned the secret and power of harmonious thought, the happy thought, the optimistic thought. They prepare their minds for a serene, harmonious night's sleep by summoning thoughts of joy, youth, peace, and love, to be their mind's guests for the night, and will entertain no others. They will not allow the old worry-thought and anxious thought to drag their hideous images through the brain to spoil their rest and leave ugly autographs in the face. The result is that they get up in the morning refreshed, rejuvenated, with all the spontaneity of their youth."

5. A hospitable mental outlook helps the nerves to get out of ruts and makes your life longer. Do we realize that in this philosophy of life and in this cultivation of an alert mental atmosphere is something of the power of the very fountain of youth? When Solon, the Athenian sage, was asked the

secret of his strength and youth, he replied that it was "learning something new every day." This belief was general among the ancient Greeks—that the secret of eternal youth was "to be always learning something new." There is a basis of truth in the idea. Says a well known physician: "It is healthful activity that strengthens and preserves the mind as well as the body, and gives it youthful quickness and activity. So, if you would be young, in spite of the years, you must remain receptive to new thought, and must grow broader in spirit, wider in sympathy and more and more open to fresh revelations of truth as you travel further on the road of life."

6. It is worth while to cultivate calmness and serenity as a fine art. "It is a great aid to the preservation of youth and vigor," says Prentice Mulford, "to be able to sit still and keep still in mind as well as in body when there is really nothing to do, because in such condition, mind and body are recuperating and filling up with new force. Do you realize that the body is not fed with material food alone? There are other elements, often unrecognized, which act upon it and give it strength, and the grand source and means of receiving these

lie partly in that mental and physical quietude of mind which acts only when it has full power to act. If wisdom guides action, either by brain or hand, a great deal more is accomplished and a balance of life's forces is kept in reserve." Do you remember what the genial doctor, Oliver Wendell Holmes, said was the secret of his marvelous youthfulness in his eightieth year? "It is due chiefly to a cheerful disposition and invariable contentment in every period of my life, with what I was. I never felt the pangs of ambition, discontent, and disquietude that makes us grow old prematurely by carving wrinkles on our faces. Wrinkles do not appear on faces that have constantly smiled. Smiling is the best possible massage. Contentment is the fountain of youth."

This trained mental outlook, therefore, is a part of the suggestion for the re-education of the nerves. In serious cases, seek a wise physician who uses both physical and psychic treatment. In milder cases, try for yourself the deliberate cultivation of cheerfulness, courage, and the great affirmations of confidence and optimism. These things will have their reaction on body—on sleep, on nerves, and on length of years.

Forel gives two excellent suggestions for

mental hygiene equally applicable to a patient passing through any nervous disorder, or to anyone desiring to keep good nervous poise. He says: "Then let the steady compass of our unswerving optimism be: Ever forward to a large-hearted ideal; never look back!" His second suggestion is "to pay as little attention as possible to functional nervous troubles and disturbances so as not to cultivate them by habit."

7. Nor must we neglect this great fact. The therapeutic value of love cannot be overestimated. As one says: "Evil thought and hateful feeling is banished by it from the mind. It tranquillizes, calms, and yet energizes the entire nature. It kindles the enthusiasm of all healthy affection and emotions. It gives a secret power that brings back and helps to maintain abounding health and unalloyed happiness. Every nerve, every muscle, every organ, feels its life-giving influence. The God of love fills His earthly temple with His hallowed presence as surely as He will fill the temple of humanity with His glory when love shall reign supreme."

Attention may be called to the fact that Ruskin dwells upon love as "the source of unity in Art, and as intimately connected with vital beauty. Through it the loveliest things are wrought. The ideal form can be reached by it alone." Leo Tolstoi strikes a fundamental note when he says: "One may deal with things without love, one may cut down trees, make bricks, and hammer iron without love, but you cannot deal with men without love."

Bishop Fallows notes that "Thomas à Kempis derived all good from love, and all evil from the opposite. He declares in his Pauline eulogy on love, 'It gives all for all, possesses all in all, because it reposes in the One Supreme Good, from which every good originates and flows.' Love is not opposed to knowledge; it is blended with it, even as it is united with faith. Reason and love ought never to come into conflict, for it would be like a house divided against itself. Let love be guided by reason and penetrated with knowledge, then will come the reconciliation of all the contradictions of life, and the harmony of mankind."

There is the remarkable case of Helen Keller, bound by physical limitations that seemed at first utterly hopeless, shut in to a world where no light nor sound ever penetrates, who has yet made such a magnificent triumph of her life that her words about joy, whose handmaid is cheerfulness, carry peculiar conviction. "Join the great company," she says, "of those who make the barren places of life fruitful with kindness. Carry a vision of heaven in your souls, and you shall make your home, your college, the world, correspond to that vision. Your success and happiness lie in you. External conditions are the accidents of life, its outer trappings. The great enduring realities are love and service. Joy is the holy fire that keeps our purpose warm and our intelligence aglow. Resolve to keep happy, and your joy and you shall form an invincible host against difficulties."

Now in all this, mental factors count for a great deal. But a more important factor than the merely mental is needed. The situation demands the fullest help, the divine and infinite background of the spiritual fellowship and power. Our chief work, if we are able, is to create a spiritual atmosphere. For this will have emphatic reaction on the physical.

1. We may remember that there is a distinct therapeutic value in a simple faith in

God. Perfect confidence in God, the rest of faith, the peace that passeth understanding, are the old phrases, which are coming to have a fuller meaning in these days.

Do you remember the word that kept the great Gladstone serene in the midst of his wearing life and heavy responsibilities? When the great burdens of his office as prime minister of England were heaviest upon him, and someone spoke to him, wondering how he could stand the terrific strain, he told the secret when he said that at the foot of his bed where he could see it when he retired, and when he rose up in the morning, were the words, "Thou wilt keep him in perfect peace whose mind is stayed on Thee, because he trusteth in Thee." Many people ought to have that verse in letters of gold where they could see it night and morning. It would put a new spirit into their lives.

As Phillips Brooks says: "Quiet has come in place of the noise; repose instead of action. . . . Some day the headlong current of your life was stopped. The river ceased to flow. The waves stood still, and then the ocean, which the flowing of the river had kept out, poured up and in, and there were sacreder emotions in the old channels, and deeper hopes and fears were beaten upon the well-worn banks. The day when your deep bereavement came, . . . the day when joy, with that subtle possibility of deep pain which is always in her eyes, came to your door and knocked, . . . the day when, being weak and ill, you did not go to your business, . . . these were the days when God was feeding you. . . . No life is complete which does not sometimes sit trustfully waiting to be fed of God."

Let me quote a letter recently received which gives a fine illustration of this process of mental and spiritual education.

It reads in part: "There came a time, after three serious illnesses, when family sorrow and responsibilities completely overtaxed me physically and mentally. I not only felt unable to go on living, but I really think my wise physician felt that I might not live if something were not done. It was then I began to seek, by God's aid, for that diviner self, which I had lost, the true and eternal 'I,' which not only could lay hold of truth, but which could detach itself utterly from the sad, weary and over-burdened individual who could not see her way to go on living. Gradually, after many failures, my consciousness of this diviner self grew stronger, recollections of old symptoms of illness became effaced from my brain and nerves, daily cares and trials ceased to affect me; my mind felt free and eager for the first time in a year to seek new truth and enjoy new beauty. And strangest of all, my strength, digestion and sleep are returning steadily. Of course I give full credit to the doctor who cured me of serious illnesses, but it was he also who urged me to a total change of thought to complete the cure."

2. Do you know that ancient but effective method, called "the practice of the presence of God?" It also has therapeutic value and is a distinct nerve tonic, as well as a life tonic.

This fine phrase of Jeremy Taylor's that haunts the soul with a continual surprise and delight is the heart of his book on "Holy Living." The book itself is an astonishment. It is so opulent in its learning, so brilliant in its phrasing, so spiritual in its feeling, and so absolutely practical in its definite counselings. It is wise in worldly wisdom, it has a flavor of colleges and king's courts and yet there is heavenly light on every page, and the pervading benediction of a splendid religious sanity. Jeremy Taylor is rightly called the Shakespeare of divines and the Chrysostom of the English Church, and his book is, "a part of that larger Bible which is the record of the deepest experiences of the most spiritual, and, therefore, the most Christian, souls of all the ages."

Says the good bishop: "We may imagine God to be in the air and the sea, and we all enclosed in His circle, wrapt up in the lap of this infinite nature. We can no more be removed from the presence of God than from our own being."

This is the general preposition which is but a phrasing of the great 139th Psalm. "Whither shall I go from Thy Spirit or whither shall I flee from Thy Presence?" Or of Paul to the Athenians: "In Him we live and move and have our being."

All of us readily admit the theory of the presence of God. It is all true, we say, and the next moment we forget it, and act as if God were far off in the infinitudes. How can we make theory into practice, how can we have God's presence so vivid and real to us as shall make it a perpetual and transforming power?

This realization of God is our own personal problem. It is the key to the art of living well, and being well. As one has rightly said, "He who realizes God will use his time aright, will have purity of motive, will be clean in thought and act, and will make his body and mind fit to be the sanctuary of the divine. . . . He who realizes God will be afraid of nothing on the earth except failing to do His will and of nothing beyond the earth except the hiding of His face."

We remember God at times and all of us realize in some measure the presence of God, but only at rare times and moments. How can we continually remember and realize God so that we shall always rejoice in Him and that He shall be continually our life and health?

If it is possible, are there any rules to compass it? Or can it be accomplished only by a great, overmastering love for God? Jeremy Taylor believed in rules as well as in love, and he gives us ten definite rules for accomplishing it in the book that we have mentioned.

Shall we venture to remind ourselves of these rules in the briefest way.

1. His first rule: Let this actual thought often return: God is omnipotent, filling

every place. "God is here." The frequent repetition of this thought will help to bring to the soul the sense of God's presence. We want the spiritual consciousness saturated with the divine reality.

2. Second rule: Solemnly worship God, place thyself in God's presence, behold Him with the eye of faith, let thy desires actually fix on Him. It is not only, "Thou God, seest me," but also "O God! I see Thee!"

3. Third rule: Let everything you see represent to you God's presence. . . . In the face of the sun you may see God's beauty; in the fire you may feel His heart warming; in the water, His gentleness to refresh you; it is the dew of heaven that makes your field give you bread and ministers drink to your necessities. This is antique imagery, but singularly suggestive. It is the spirit of the higher pantheism to which Saint Francis of Assisi gives utterance in his childlike yet majestic "Hymn of the Creatures."

4. Fourth rule: Make frequent short discoursings between God and thy own soul. This will make Him present to thy spirit and to thy necessity. This was long since called by a spiritual person "A building to God a chapel in our breast." For thus in the midst

of your work, you may retire into your chapel—your heart—and converse with God.

5. Fifth rule: "Express thyself constantly, sensible of God by a spirit of love and reverence toward Him." God is present by His power, He calls for reverence; He is present to Thee in Thy needs and relieves them; He deserves Thy love.

6. Sixth rule: "Remember God is in us, we are in Him." We are in His actual presence by His indwelling within us, and by our partaking of His divine nature. Let this thought make Him real to us. It is the spirit of Novalis, "Whoso toucheth my flesh, toucheth God."

7. Seventh rule: "God is in thy brother. Refresh Him when he needs it." Thou givest to thy brother, thou givest to God, for He is thy brother. This is the ancient word of Christ and this the modern parable of Sir Launfal.

8. Eighth rule: "Everywhere let your deportment be as if in a holy place," or on holy ground, for God is there. God is in this place though I may know it not . . . this is a gate of heaven.

9. Ninth rule: "Remember that God is in every creature. Be cruel toward none."

Be kind toward all, for it is God who is in all by His presence. Almost there seems here the exquisite sense of sanctity of the Buddhists, and the closing lesson of the rhyme of the Ancient Mariner.

10. Tenth rule: "Companion thyself with God. . . . Converse with Him, run to Him in all thy necessities; ask counsel of Him in all thy doubtings; weep before Him for thy sins; fear Him as a judge, reverence Him as a lord, obey Him as a father, love Him . . . as the espoused loves his betrothed."

These are the Ten Rules for the practice of the presence of God, and the rules are supplemented by a number of excellent prayers to be used in furtherance of the practice.

Notice in all these rules that the way of realization is not when we minimize self; not in the ascetic sense of effacing personality and nullifying will, but in the sense of finding the larger life, by forgetting self and remembering God.

Tolstoi is correct, as Dr. MacDonald remarks, when he said the cause of all our ills is that men have lost their sense of God. That is why we rush at our brother's throat;

that is why we struggle and compete, and claw and cheat, and lose our life more and more with every futile attempt to save it. Yes, and that is the cause of our sorrows, our sicknesses and our despair. We have refused to believe that God is with us and that we are spirits as infinite as is He; and that because spirit with spirit can meet, the very joy of heaven is at our door waiting to be brought up into our consciousness and made the working principle of existence.

Such great truths—when we meditate upon them often, repeat them over and over again until we live with them and they become a part of us—cannot fail to bring a more joyous and confident mind and spirit, and react most helpfully and hopefully on the whole life—spiritually, mentally, even physically.

Such things we must emphasize.

We need to make it our habit to realize the presence of God, of the omnipresence of His goodness, His wisdom, His love and His power with us. We need to keep constantly before us in all our daily life, the remembrance that it is in God that we live and move and have our being. We need to speak frequently to all the troubles, disturbances and worries of life, "In the name of Christ, peace, be still!"

Then from words we can go to facts. For it is actual fact that God is within us; we can be one with Him. We can possess the divine presence; it possesses us. We can come into fuller and fuller realization that the transcendent God is also an immanent God in the depths of the life. We can learn in prayer and communion to withdraw from the consciousness of the morbid and painful, at least for some quiet hours in the midst of the day—withdraw into the consciousness of the divine and eternal. Just as one can forget pain in a great joy, or forget time and place in an absorbing story, or forget all as the eyes close and sleep comes —so can we sink into God in restfulness and peace, and awake to new strength and health.

Is this mysticism? It is also practicality. It is not a life of mere passivity and acquiescence, but of positiveness and action. It means incitement toward strongest personality. It is letting God work through you to the fullest. It is asserting independence in spiritual things under the leadership of the Spirit. It is standing on one's feet with

God and emphasizing the reality and supremacy of the spiritual in life. It is facing all the circumstances of life with the cry, "I conquer in Christ. I can do all things through Him." It is being grateful for the stimulus of hardness and attack. It is meeting trials, troubles, suffering and sadness—and searching their very depths until the heart of blessing in them is found. It is living in the turmoils and struggles and battles of life with the deep hidden serenity of God at the heart, like the calm in the deep ocean caves though the upper surface be storm. It is making the very best of life. The conditions of life may be hard, hostile and harassing. But what of it? We can never reach our ideal conditions. We must realize that where we are and in our present conditions, life's discipline must be endured and conquered and life's divinest lessons learned.

Such things as these we must emphasize. God is near us now and here, as if we were with Him in Heaven.

The Almighty is right here—in us—abounding, infinite in His wisdom and love and power for us. The power of the Almighty is for us and for our using. Just as much as we can use worthily and well, not for ecstasy, not for display, but for spiritual service—so much is God eager and willing to give us. It is ours if we will be filled with all the fullness of God.

We must emphasize above all, what is the vital center of life. Shall we dwell in the trivialities of self, of fears and doubts and weakness, and frailties and sickness, of things that are accidental, temporary, that perish with the using—shall we make these the all-important things of life? Or shall we dwell on the eternal things—of truth, of character, of God and His love, and His promises, and holiness and health? Once it was thought that this earth was the center of the universe and all things else revolved around it. The universe was geo-centric. That was Ptolamaic astronomy. But we have learned better since Copernicus, and it is seen that the sun is the center and all revolves around it. The universe, as we know it, is helio-centric.

Perchance we have been making our own little selves too much the center of our thought, care, interest, religion. We have lost power and peace. God calls us to let our lives be not self-centered. He wants our thought, love, interests, hopes, all to revolve around the Son of God. In Him is holiness and health.

Do we understand, and are we helping others to understand, what it means to live in an atmosphere of large inspiration? It comes by dwelling in the great affirmations of divine truth, the eternal verities of existence. And do we realize how such a divine atmosphere can remake the whole life, physical, as well as mental and moral?

The Master said, eighteen hundred years ago, "Have faith in God"; the Psalmist said a thousand years or more before that, "Hope thou in God." Implicit trust in God —believing love—is the true philosopher's stone that transmutes everything that it touches into gold, that takes these rough, bitter experiences of life and sees them full of the golden goodness of God. "Believing love!" It is the fabled maiden that goes forth weaving with a magic web. She snatches here and there the scattered skeins of this tangled universe and weaves them together as silken threads, into one glorious, harmonious garment of the goodness of God.

The only thing that makes serious and intelligent men live content and hopeful in the midst of the mysterious and oftentimes bitter and perplexing providences of life, is this firm assurance, that behind this world and its mysteries there is One whose name is love, One who loves us heart to heart, One who is manifesting His love to us in a thousand ways. He is the clew of the maze; He is the center and heart of the world's life and purposes; His is the plan and consummation of that

> ". . . one far-off divine event,
> To which the whole creation moves."

BEST BOOKS

FOR FURTHER READING

BEST BOOKS FOR FURTHER READING

1. ON THE GENERAL SUBJECT.

Rational Living—Pres. Henry Churchill King.

Methods and Problems of Spiritual Healing—Prof. Horatio W. Dresser.

Religion and Medicine—Drs. Elwood Worcester, Samuel McComb, Isador H. Coriat.

The Will to be Well—Charles Brodie Patterson.

Work and Mind—Dr. Luther H. Gulick.

The Quest of Health and Happiness—Rev. Chauncey R. Hawkins.

Health Through Self-Control—William Anthony Spinney.

Power Through Repose and *The Freedom of Life*—Annie Payson Call

How to Get Strong—Prof. John S. Blaikie.

Ideal Suggestion, Through Mental Photography—Henry Wood.

Why Worry?—Charles Walton, M. D.

Health and Happiness—Bishop Samuel Fallows.

Mind, Religion and Health—Rev. Robert MacDonald, D. D.

What All the World's A-Seeking, and *In Tune With the Infinite*—Ralph Waldo Trine.

Every Man a King—Orison S. Marden.

Mind Power and Privileges—Albert B. Olston.

Paths to the Heights—Dr. Sheldon Leavitt.
Menticulture—Horace Fletcher.
The Victory of the Will—Victor Charbounel.
Energies of Man—Prof. William James.

2. ON THE MEDICAL ASPECTS.

The Psychic Treatment of Nervous Disorders—Dr. Paul DuBois.
Psychotherapy and its Relation to Medicine—Richard C. Cabot, M. D.
Doctor and Patient—S. Weir Mitchell, M. D.
Self-Help for Nervous Women—John K. Mitchell, M. D.
On the Obscure Diseases of the Brain and Disorders of the Mind—Forbes Winslow, M. D.
American Nervousness, its Causes and Consequences—Dr. George M. Beard.
Hypnotism and Psychotherapy—Forel.
Demon Possession and Allied Themes—Nevius.
Lectures on Clinical Psychiatry—Dr. Emil Kraepelin.
The Force of Mind, Unconscious Therapeutics, and *Nerves in Disorder*—Dr. Alfred T. Schofield.
Hypnotism, its History, Practice and Theory—Dr. J. Milne Bramwell.

3. ON THE PSYCHOLOGICAL ASPECTS.

Psychology—Prof. William James.
Outlines of Psychology—Prof. Josiah Royce.
Mental Development, its Methods and Processes—Prof. Mark Baldwin.
The Influence of Mind on Body—Dr. Paul DuBois.

BOOKS FOR FURTHER READING

Physiological Psychology—Prof. W. Wundt.

The Subconscious Self and its Relation to Education and Health—Dr. Louis Waldstein.

The Subconscious—Prof. Jastrow.

Psychology and Life, and *Psychotherapy*—Prof. Hugo Munsterberg.

Psychology and Common Life—Dr. Hoffman.

The Psychology of Jesus—A. W. Hitchcock.

The Religious Aspect of Philosophy—Prof. Josiah Royce.

Multiple Personality—Dr. Boris Sidis.

Human Personality and its Survival of Bodily Death—F. W. H. Myers.

The Philosophy of the Unconscious—Edouard Von Hartmann.

Spiritual Consciousness—Frank H. Sprague.

The Varieties of Religious Experience and *Talks to Teachers on Psychology*—Prof. William James.

The Dissociation of a Personality—Dr. Morton Prince.

Adolescence, its Psychology—Prof. G. Stanley Hall.

Psychic Research and Gospel Miracles—Rev. E. M. Hoff and Thomas G. Allen, M. D.

Made in the USA
Monee, IL
04 November 2026

67385023R00144